25 Natural Ways to Manage Stress and Prevent Burnout

Also by James Scala, Ph.D.:

Arthritis: Diet Against It
The High Blood Pressure Relief Diet
If You Can't/Won't Stop Smoking
Making the Vitamin Connection
The New Arthritis Relief Diet
The New Eating Right for a Bad Gut
Prescription for Longevity

25 Natural Ways to Manage Stress and Prevent Burnout

A MIND-BODY APPROACH TO HEALTH AND WELL-BEING

James Scala, Ph.D.

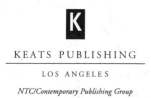

KEATS PUBLISHING

LOS ANGELES

NTC/Contemporary Publishing Group

Library of Congress Cataloging-in-Publication Data

Scala, James, 1934-
    25 natural ways to manage stress and prevent burnout : a mind-body approach to health and well-being / James Scala.
      p. cm.
    Includes index.
    ISBN 0-658-00700-9
    1. Stress (Psychology) 2. Stress management. I. Title: Twenty-five natural ways to manage stress and prevent burnout. II. Title.

BF575.S75 S33 2000
155.9'042—dc21

                                00-043402

Published by Keats Publishing
A division of NTC/Contemporary Publishing Group, Inc.
4255 West Touhy Avenue, Lincolnwood, Illinois 60646-1975 U.S.A.

Managing Director and Publisher: Jack Artenstein
Executive Editor: Peter Hoffman
Director of Publishing Services: Rena Copperman
Managing Editor: Jama Carter
Editor: Claudia McCowan
Project Editor: Judith Liggett

Text design by Wendy Staroba Loreen

Printed in the United States of America

International Standard Book Number: 0-658-00700-9

00 01 02 03 04 DHD 15 14 13 12 11 10 9 8 7 6 5 4 3 2 1

Contents

Introduction

THE STRESS EPIDEMIC

During the twentieth century, life expectancy at birth almost doubled, from the low forties in 1900 to almost seventy by 1996. Comparing the most common causes of death in 1900 to those in 1996 provides insight into what twentieth-century technology has accomplished in terms of health, for both better and worse.

As listed in Table I.1, communicable diseases were the three most common causes of death in 1900; in 1996, diet and stress-related diseases accounted for the four most common causes. Diabetes, suicide, chronic liver disease, and accidents all have dietary and stress connections as well. As the twentieth century came to a close, seven of the top ten causes of death were significantly influenced, if not caused, by stress. Stress is inarguably on the rise, and as stress increases, our health suffers.

The Relationship Between Stress and Disease

Stress causes or influences all the diseases listed in Table I.1 through its effect on our diet and lifestyle habits. A person who can't control stress in a healthy way uses alternative stress relievers, such as smoking, or omits beneficial activities, such as exercise, to alleviate its

Table I.1

Most Common Causes of Death

Rank	1900 Cause	1996 Cause
1	Pneumonia and influenza	Heart disease
2	Tuberculosis	Cancer
3	Diarrhea and enteritis	Stroke
4	Heart disease	Pulmonary diseases
5	Brain hemorrhage (stroke)	Accidents
6	Kidney disease	Pneumonia and influenza
7	Accidents	Diabetes
8	Cancer	AIDS
9	Senility*	Suicide
10	Diphtheria	Chronic liver disease

*Possibly Alzheimer's disease, first diagnosed in 1906.

symptoms. These negative habits are not always obvious stress relievers, nor are they obvious causes of fatal disease. Compare the health problems they produce, listed below, to the modern causes of death listed in Table I.1.

Each of the health problems listed in the chart on page xiii creates additional health problems, because each one complicates other diseases, many of which become apparent only as we age. For example, as people grow older, their bone calcium becomes depleted and they can develop osteoporosis. The risk of osteoporosis can be reduced by taking calcium supplements, but it is made worse by smoking, excessive alcohol intake, stimulants, incorrect food choices, and inadequate exercise—all of which are common stress relievers. The relationship between stress and osteoporosis is so indirect, however, that neither the sixty-five-year-old with osteoporosis nor her doctor will ever relate the disease to the lifetime of stress that preceded its onset.

We can expect our lives to be ever more enriched, and ever more complicated, by the marvels of technology, so we must face the dark

Stress Relievers That Detract from Health	
Stress Relievers	**Related Health Problems**
Overeating	Cardiovascular disease
Smoking	Diabetes (adult onset or Type 2)
Alcohol	High blood pressure
High-fat foods	Cancer
Excessively sweet foods	Liver disease
Salty foods and snacks	Kidney disease
Poor exercise habits	Lung disease

side of progress and learn to deal with the stress it has helped to create. We must learn to cope with the myriad options the modern world offers in careers, lifestyles, entertainment, and so forth. We're often faced with more choices than we can effectively understand, let alone use efficiently. The complexity of modern life often means we have to do several things at once, each of which used to be done as individual activities.

The tips in this handy book help you deal with the stress that accompanies the abundance of our world today.

UNDERSTANDING HOW STRESS WORKS

The word *stress* has a personal meaning for each of us. We live in an age of anxiety in which just about everyone experiences some level of stress from pressures brought on by a complex, competitive, not always supportive society. Technically, stress is the actual bodily wear and tear caused by these pressures, which we'll call *stressors*.

Stress isn't necessarily a bad thing. An athlete in training methodically and purposefully stresses her body so it will rise to a higher level of performance and the athletic event will not exhaust her. Other examples of using stress to one's advantage include the practice sessions of police and firefighters, and the everyday exercise many of us do to stay fit. Planned physical stress, such as sensible exercise, can improve our capacity to handle both physical and emotional stress.

To most of us, however, stress means the everyday emotional challenges we face that take a toll on our health and general well-being. We've all overheard the comment, "He's getting gray too soon," or "She looks older than her age." Worse yet is the comment, "Well, he was under a lot of stress;" we often hear this said about someone who has had a heart attack.

How we deal with all stress, physical and mental, is based on the "fight-or-flight" capability. This is what equips our bodies to meet a clear, dangerous physical challenge. In the face of more subtle emotional challenges, however, it can do more harm than good.

The Fight-or-Flight Response: Physical Stress

You're walking on a lonely street at night when a man jumps out from a doorway. In an instant you tense up and either start running or stand and fight. The attacker is a clear challenge—technically, a well-defined stressor. Your autonomic nervous system (which doesn't include your brain) puts your body into fight-or-flight mode without any conscious thought on your part. Several very important changes take place in the instant you are confronted by the attacker:

- Digestion stops dead. This enables your blood to be directed to your muscles, so you can run or fight, and to your brain, so you can think quickly.
- Your breathing quickens even before you start running or fighting, bringing more oxygen to your lungs which, in turn increases the transfer of oxygen to your blood.
- Your heart rate (pulse) increases rapidly, raising your blood

pressure. The oxygen-rich blood is pumped more rapidly to your muscles and brain, enabling heightened energy production.

- Sweating starts instantly. This dissipates body heat caused by the increased blood flow and energy you're about to expend.
- Muscles tense for action, making you ready to run or fight. Tense muscles are also better able to withstand physical force, such as a blow or knife wound.
- Clotting chemicals pour into your blood to ensure that bleeding stops quickly if you are injured so you can keep going.
- Energy-yielding glucose (blood sugar) is released into the blood for quick energy, and fat is released to provide prolonged energy in case you have to keep running or fighting.

An attack is a clear example of a stressful event—pretty much what a caveman would have faced many eons ago if he encountered a wild animal. These physiological processes are a deeply ingrained part of our genetic makeup.

Physical stress causes your body to produce the hormones norepinephrine (in large quantity) and epinephrine (in modest quantity), which together are called adrenaline. Adrenaline causes the increase in heart rate, blood flow, and blood pressure that enables the fight-or-flight response. Athletes warm up before a contest or workout to get their adrenaline flowing, which prepares their bodies for the upcoming ordeal.

Emotional Stress

You're working in an understaffed, competitive marketing department. Project demands keep piling up, your "in box" is full, the "out box" is glaringly empty, and your computer is so clogged with e-mail the hard drive is gagging. You're bucking for a promotion; you want the title, plush office, and secretary; and most of all, you need the money to pay off your maxed-out credit cards and the braces your daughter needs. On top of that, you must attend many unproductive meetings and report to management about your projects that need attention and work, as if just reporting problems will somehow fix them. You've noticed a few disturbing things about yourself in these meetings:

- You get butterflies in your stomach. You often skip lunch afterward or get something from a vending machine and make do with a cup of coffee. Sometimes you even think about trying a cigarette.
- You feel almost out of breath when a vice president poses a probing question and you don't have the good, simple, optimistic answer he really wants.
- Your heart often seems to pound when you're on the spot. You notice that sometimes your chest seems a little tight, even if the feeling passes quickly.
- Recently you purchased an antiperspirant that's advertised to "dry up an ocean" because your armpits are always getting wet, calling for costly dry cleaning. Ironically, the office temperature is usually somewhat cool.
- You often feel yourself filling with anger, but quickly suppress the feeling; outwardly you are the picture of calm, while inwardly you are uptight.
- Coworkers often tell you not to speak so loudly, when you hadn't realized you had raised your voice.

In addition, you have noticed some disturbing after-work tendencies:

- At home in the evening, you often have a stiff neck and the muscles in your lower back are tight.
- You feel tired at night, but usually bring work home and are

still at it after your spouse is asleep. And when you do go to bed, you have trouble falling asleep.

- If you're a man, you often can't perform as well sexually as you used to perform. If you're a woman, you find you simply aren't interested.

The release of both adrenaline and another hormone, cortisol, is triggered by emotional stress. Cortisol prepares us for vigorous physical activity by releasing reserves of energy substances such as protein, fat, and glycogen held in lean tissue for conversion to glucose as an additional prolonged energy source. Prolonged physical activity burns off the results of this hormonal rush. In emotionally stressful situations, the blood glucose and fatty acids are released, not burned off. Generally, we don't leave stressful meetings or family arguments and go get a good workout to burn off these chemicals; instead, we might go to a business lunch, have a drink or a cup of coffee, or simply sulk. Each option leaves the body with a serious problem: elevated blood chemicals that under more "primitive" conditions would have been dissipated by physical activity.

Two insidious by-products of prolonged cortisol elevation are increased stomach acidity and lean tissue breakdown. Therefore, prolonged emotional stress leads to ulcers and a weakened body, causing your muscle strength to actually decline. That's why stress and ulcers seem to go together; ulcers are the result of stress that has no other outlet.

Physical and Emotional Stress: Is There a Difference?

The primitive fight-or-flight response is alive and well in the modern environment. These seemingly different instances of physical and emotional stress actually have many similarities to those of ancient times. They are almost identical in the short-term effects they have on the body. Even though you work in an office, drive a bus, or are a night-shift nurse, your body responds to challenges just as it would have 10,000 years ago in a camp attacked by looters. Instead of picking up a spear, throwing a rock, or running and hiding, however, you have to hide your emotions, you can't run, and if you raise your voice or show anger you'll soon go to the unemployment line. As you cover up all these biochemical changes that stress triggers, they simmer beneath the surface and slowly take a toll on your health—unless you take steps to dissipate their effects and prevent them from happening in the first place.

THE EFFECTS OF STRESS OVER TIME

Humans are nothing if not adaptable. Not only can we adapt to almost any climate, we can adapt and survive the extremes of all kinds of physical and mental duress.

While the biochemical effects of physical stressors are usually modulated, the effects of emotional stress are not dissipated; in fact, they're made worse by the most common stress relievers, which are themselves often stressors. These include excesses of caffeine, alcohol, and calories, and other things such as smoking. The most common stress reliever is snacking; as if the excess calories weren't bad enough, too often the least healthy food is selected.

Emotionally stressful confrontations, particularly those at work, are often scheduled so the participants can deal with difficult issues and then have a nice meal afterward. Worse yet, tough meetings are often followed by a stop at the nearest bar or cocktail lounge to "let go." People often give bad news in public—such as at lunch—so that the recipient is too embarrassed to become "emotional." The tradition of "breaking bread" to make peace is deeply rooted in most cultures. In our modern world, however, it would be best to go to the nearest gym and have a good forty-minute workout, or take a brisk forty-minute walk through the park, rather than eat a meal.

Extreme Reactions to Physical and Emotional Stress

The fight-or-flight response causes an increase in blood pressure, heart rate, and blood-clotting factors, as well as elevated blood sugar and fat—all risk factors for a stroke or heart attack. Any doctor who finds these factors elevated in a patient's annual physical is ethically obligated to advise him to get started on a proper diet and a sensible exercise program, and in some cases to prescribe appropriate medication to normalize blood chemistry.

A person who suffers from extreme emotional stress is making herself vulnerable to heart attack or stroke. How many times have you heard about a person who had a heart attack when confronted by a burglar or while shoveling snow? When an executive, young or old, has a heart attack or stroke, talk seems to turn immediately to the pressure he was under at work. At one time or another, everyone resolves to "take things a little less seriously," but how many really follow through? Following are common risk factors for stroke and heart attack:

- Elevated blood pressure
- Elevated blood fat including cholesterol
- Elevated blood sugar
- Excess weight, especially abdominal weight
- Elevated pulse rate

A Clear Price

When stress is imposed regularly on someone who doesn't recognize what is happening or doesn't take steps to prevent or deal well with it, a severe price is paid. The most common health problems caused by regular stress are:

- Elevated blood pressure (hypertension)
- Elevated blood sugar (Type 2 diabetes)

- Elevated blood fat (triglycerides), including cholesterol, the major risk factors for cardiovascular disease
- Ulcers in the stomach and small intestine
- Serious weight gain or, rarely, serious weight loss
- Increased susceptibility to diseases

Emotional health suffers as well. While regular exercise can train the body to deal with physical stress and can help normalize blood chemistry, our mental reactions are often left hanging. The brain, like any organ, must be trained to deal with stress. If we don't train it sensibly and follow a good diet, our emotional health suffers and can produce:

- Overreactions to minor stressors
- Difficulty interacting calmly with others
- Inability to empathize with others
- Reduced ability to accept new situations
- Incorrect, usually negative, perceptions of change
- Increased susceptibility to emotional disorders

REDUCING AND MANAGING STRESS

We can deal with stress in three ways:

1. Manage stressors and make sure they are held to a minimum level.
2. Exercise mentally and physically, so that the effects of stress can be faced down or dissipated.
3. Eat correctly and use supplements sensibly, so that unavoidable stress cannot exert lasting effects on health.

This book discusses these three approaches to stress relief, identifying ways you can manage or reduce stress.

1

Determine Just How Stressed You Are

Stress levels change. We all go through times when life is not just good, it's great; for example, a two-week vacation at a resort where your toughest decision is choosing what you'll have for dinner, or times at work when things just seem to fall into place and you get the recognition you deserve. But there are also the times when the hot water runs out just as you get in the shower, the coffeemaker decides to quit, and there is an accident that causes a major traffic jam on your way to work.

Our lives are not consistent. Without some stress they'd be dull, but with too much, we get ulcers. Can we evaluate the amount of stress in our lives to see if it's at a healthy level? The answer is yes!

THE STRESS TEST

Stress is often about change; how often you must adjust to some event or events determines, in part, your degree of stress. A bad commute is stressful, but if it occurs only once in a while, you can get over it. If it is every day and you don't do something to eliminate the stress (for example, take the train rather than drive as you usually do), you have to adjust. We can adjust only so much before this starts taking a toll on our health. Scientists have devised a social readjustment test that quantifies how much we have had to adjust in the past year.

Before You Take the Test

- You will notice that the questions are all about personal relationships. Most stress comes from our dealings with others.
- Most questions are about change. Humans can adjust to almost any situation if it is consistent and not too many changes are needed.
- Some questions focus on good things (for example, winning the lottery). When we get a windfall it changes our lives and we must adjust once again.
- If you had taken the test six months ago, you would have had a different score. If you take it six months from now, your score will again be different. As the demands placed on us change, so do our levels of stress.

Now take the test.

The Test

When reviewing the test, you'll notice that some questions ask about things that are only slightly different; for example, purchasing a house versus remodeling a house. Do your best to keep such events distinct. However, do interpret when appropriate; for example, if you experienced the death of a *very* close friend who meant as much to you as a family member does, answer the question about family members rather than the question about close friends.

Score each event according to the number of times it has happened in the last twelve months. It is often helpful to have a close friend or family member help you with these questions. You will get a much more realistic and objective answer.

The Stress Test

Life Event	Stress Value	x	Number of times you experienced it this year	=	Total Score
Death of a spouse, child, or significant other	100		_____		_____
Divorce or breakup of a long-standing (two years or more) cohabitating relationship	73		_____		_____
Separation without divorce	65		_____		_____
Detention, jail, medical institutionalization, or legal restriction, such as with visitation rights	63		_____		_____
Death of a family member	63		_____		_____
Major injury or illness or serious corrective surgery	53		_____		_____
Marriage or decision to cohabitate	50		_____		_____
Losing your job, firing, layoff (not your choice)	47		_____		_____
Marital reconciliation with mate or significant other	45		_____		_____
Retirement because of age or request (not your choice)	45		_____		_____

The Stress Test (continued)

Life Event	Stress Value	x	Number of times you experienced it this year	=	Total Score
Health change or behavioral change in family member	44		_____		_____
Pregnancy (both partners)	40		_____		_____
Sexual dysfunction (vaginal dryness, loss of desire)	39		_____		_____
Family gain: birth, adoption, older child moves back, parent moves in, foster child, acquiring a significant pet	39		_____		_____
Major business change: merger, bankruptcy, move to new location with difficult change in commute	39		_____		_____
Major change in financial status (lose a lot of money in stock market, are swindled, win lottery, gain big inheritance)	38		_____		_____
Death of a close friend or an important long-term pet	37		_____		_____
A major career change or line of work change	36		_____		_____

The Stress Test (continued)

Life Event	Stress Value	x	Number of times you experienced it this year	=	Total Score
Change in spousal or relationship with significant other (for example, many arguments or no more arguments)	35		_____		_____
Taking on a significant financial obligation: house mortgage, business loan, home-improvement loan	31		_____		_____
Foreclosure on a loan	30		_____		_____
Major change in work status: big promotion, demotion, lateral transfer, someone else is promoted	29		_____		_____
Son or daughter leaves home (for college, marriage, military)	29		_____		_____
In-law problems, including live-in partnerships	29		_____		_____
Outstanding personal achievement (Pulitzer or other academic prize, employee of year, player of the year)	28		_____		_____

The Stress Test (continued)

Life Event	Stress Value	x	Number of times you experienced it this year	=	Total Score
Spouse (or significant other) going to work outside home or quitting work outside home	28		___		___
Schooling: beginning or stopping formal schooling essential to your career	26		___		___
Major change in present living conditions: building a new home, serious remodel of present home, deterioration of present home (fire, earthquake, roof collapse) or neighborhood goes bad (prostitutes or gangs move in)	24		___		___
Forced change of dress habits: you're formal, now it's casual or vice versa	24		___		___
Boss is causing trouble: doesn't like you, is not nice	23		___		___
Major change in working conditions: from flex time to a strict nine to five, night work, from office or cubicle to sharing a large office with many co-workers	20		___		___
Move to new residence, but keep same job	20		___		___

The Stress Test (continued)

Life Event	Stress Value	x	Number of times you experienced it this year	=	Total Score
Change in recreation (give up tennis or start tennis; start exercise program or stop exercising)	19		_____		_____
Change in religious activities (start, stop, join a new group)	19		_____		_____
Social or service club change: join, drop out, take on a new role	18		_____		_____
Loan for large expenses (car, pool, country club fee)	17		_____		_____
Sleeping habits change (you used to sleep 7 hours each night and now you sleep 2 hours more or 2 hours less)	16		_____		_____
Family gatherings change: many more, many less (include extended family)	15		_____		_____
Eating habits change: eat more or less; change to new variety (become vegetarian or quit being vegetarian and eat meat)	15		_____		_____
Vacation	13		_____		_____

The Stress Test (continued)

Life Event	Stress Value	x	Number of times you experienced it this year	=	Total Score
Christmas	12		_____		_____
Minor legal problems: traffic tickets, disturbing the peace	11		_____		_____

Reprinted from the *Journal for Psychosomatic Research*, Vol. 11, Holmes and Rehs, "The Social Readjustment Rating Scale," 1967. Used with permission from Elsevier Science.

Scoring

What does your score say about you and your life? The higher your score, the greater your stress level. However, a low score is not necessarily always good, because boredom is stressful in itself.

- *300 or above:* You have been forced to make many serious adjustments. A high score is correlated to more illness, injury, accidents, and other preventable problems and events in all walks of life; for example, a professional athlete with such a high score would be more likely to be injured in a game; similarly, a delivery person could have an accident, such as hitting a pedestrian. It suggests you are troubled by major events in your life and you could drop your guard. If you don't plan to make some changes to reduce the tempo of your readjustment, at least take out a larger life insurance policy.
- *150 to 300:* You're in the moderate range and you've been living a hassled life. Review the sources of your score. If it is a lot of onetime events, you can probably be confident that if you take the test in six months, you'll score in the normal (50 to 150) range. If your score is due to reoccurring events, you should start a serious program to eliminate stressors or hassles in your life.
- *50 to 150:* You're like the rest of us. Life is a challenge and you are probably meeting its challenges. If you feel stressed and you've taken the test honestly, you could be expecting too much. Look to this or other books, or perhaps to a counselor, to help you adjust to the normal pace of life.
- *50 or below:* If you feel stress, it is from boredom. Boredom is stressful; in fact, it can be dangerous. This doesn't mean you're a boring person, but it indicates you need more

activities in your life that involve other people. Carefully assess your interests (gardening, music, art, and so on) and seek out organizations that reflect those interests. If you've always wanted to do something challenging (bungee jumping, working for a good cause), you could probably benefit by doing it (within reason).

2

Keep a Stress Diary

Whenever someone I know is thinking of changing jobs, I always tell him or her to write down the "reasons for" and "reasons against" the present job and the proposed or future job. Writing things down on paper is a way of removing them from ourselves and putting them at arm's length. We can see things objectively, without emotion.

Stress is no different! It can be managed only if it is put on the table, free of emotion, and its means of elimination or control identified. If there are no obvious means of elimination or control, then you must learn to externalize it and keep it from affecting you.

The first step in eliminating stress is to figure out when you are usually stressed. If your stress is related to work, is it during or after certain meetings, during your commute, or when you're around specific people? If you find that you're stressed at home, is it when your children behave defiantly, or when your spouse acts indifferently toward you?

Your objective is clear: realistically identify those things that make your life difficult on a regular basis. We all have occasional stress, but ongoing stress in particular must be managed.

IDENTIFY THE SOURCE OF YOUR STRESS

Once you know when you're stressed, you can identify the source. It is not enough to say, for instance, "The weekly marketing report meeting always makes me stressed"; you've got to identify some specifics: "The sales VP always finds something awry in my cost analysis," or "The sales VP pays no attention to my report."

MAKE A PLAN OF ACTION

Once you have identified the source of your stress, you can identify an action plan that will neutralize it. For example, if you find your-self saying:

- "The sales VP always finds something awry in my cost analysis at meetings," then sit down with that person and ask, "What do you look for in a cost analysis?" Get back to basics and find out why he wants that information; you'll learn how to make his day. Or suppose he just likes giving you a hard time: you can choose to let it run off your back, use humor to deal with him, or find a way of making his motivation obvious to your coworkers. With a little thought and effort, you've converted that stressful meeting to one that you can live with, if not enjoy.
- "My thirteen-year-old daughter wants to wear makeup to school against my wishes," then ask yourself, is it really reasonable to expect your daughter to fight peer pressure completely? Is this a chance to teach a lesson in moderation? A chance to gain her confidence? Set some reasonable guidelines—for instance, saying that moderate lipstick is okay, but no eye makeup—that you both might find acceptable.

YOUR STRESS DIARY

Purchase a bound, lined notebook, conveniently sized so you can carry it with you if necessary. Quality is important; choose something durable so you can go back, say, six months from now, and see how far you've come. On the left page, summarize the stressor in general terms in about two or three sentences, the shorter the better. On the right page, write the manifestation of your stress; in short, how the stressor is making life difficult for you. On the left page below the original paragraph, write the problem. On the right page opposite the problem, write the solution (or a possible solution).

Take this example from Ray's diary:

Stressor: Bored to death during my daily commute . . . and feel guilty. (This represents two problems: Ray's bored and he feels guilty about the wasted time.)

Manifestation: Sleep has become a way of dealing with my problems. For example, if I sit down to read a paper or a good book, I fall asleep. I even find myself nodding off during meetings.

Problem: I can't avoid the commute because I can't afford to live in New York City.

Solution: Use commuting time to learn an entirely new trade so I can get out of this mess and work at home.

Ray bought books and tapes on jewelry and jewelry making. In the evenings and on Saturdays he started creating jewelry and became good at it. Eventually this hobby turned into a profession. By working at home as a jeweler, he was able to say good-bye to commuting and turn stress into a new career.

3

Establish Your Priorities

Want to live in the British Virgin Islands? It's terrific there. The weather is always great, the water's clear, people are relaxed, and there is always a cool breeze. If living there is your first priority, however, you'd better not plan on a career in the computer industry unless it involves selling computers to the few people there who need them.

Priorities, often not our own, shape our lives. Our religion, politics, attitudes, interests, and morals are often shaped by our parents' priorities. As we grow older and learn about life, we start choosing our priorities. Setting good priorities in life is critical because each choice has trade-offs; each one carries a price.

For instance, if you absolutely must live in an urban area, you have set a serious priority. The city might offer excellent cultural opportunities, unbelievable beauty within easy reach, and excellent universities. At the same time, getting around in a busy metropolis can be a nightmare, the schools may not be very good, and urban living takes a lot of money! In contrast, if you're willing to live elsewhere, say, in a nearby suburb, you can look forward to much cheaper housing, easier commutes if you work locally, better educational options, and generally lower living costs.

HOW TO ESTABLISH PRIORITIES

Each of us has a set of priorities in life. A worthwhile exercise is to approach these priorities the following way:

- Imagine yourself dying on your one hundredth birthday. One of your great-great-grandchildren is told to write a one-page obituary about you. Write that obituary, assuming you've accomplished everything important to you.
- Imagine you're sixty-five years old and your high school reunion is coming up. Your former classmates must receive a one-page essay of what you've done with your life. Write that essay.

Now do the following:

- List the ten most important things you want to accomplish in the next decade. Rank them in order of importance.
- List the ten most important things you want to accomplish in the next five years.
- List the ten most important things you want to accomplish in the next year.
- List the ten most important things you want to accomplish in the next six months.
- List the ten most important things you want to accomplish in the next month.
- List the ten most important things you want to accomplish tomorrow.

Do those priorities telescope into each other? How? How do they stack up against your imagined obituary? Your reunion essay?

If they don't all telescope together somehow, you'd better reevaluate your priorities. If you don't, you can expect an increasingly stressful life with constantly increasing conflicts.

If you have a family, have your family members do the same exercise. You might notice lots of disconnected priorities. Now might be a good time to get family priorities into harmony.

Well-established priorities are also important in the world of work. Everyone in the company must have priorities that mesh with one another. The best question you can ask of yourself and your coworkers at the close of a business meeting is simple: "What are our priorities for tomorrow in view of what we did today?"

PRIORITIZE DAILY TASKS

Take a few quiet moments at the beginning of each day to set and assess that day's goals. Prioritize these goals, because you're unlikely to get to all of them. Set them in the wrong order and you'll be under lots of stress. The people with the most stress are those who cannot prioritize their goals or even their daily tasks. If they see a list of ten "to do's," they give each one equal weight. That is an invitation to internal mental stress for various reasons; for instance, stress from working overly long hours or stress from disintegrating interpersonal relationships because there's never time for fun.

DAILY AFFIRMATION

Start each day by reaffirming your personal and professional priorities. Set aside five minutes and do it in a quiet place by yourself where nothing else is happening. This allows you to reset your basic compass on a daily basis.

Think back briefly to that imagined one hundredth birthday, or the "what I did with my life" composition. There is always time to do better; let it start in this five-minute affirmation.

TIME OUTS

Each day will present unexpected challenges. How you deal with them will not only eventually define who you are, but also affect those around you. When a crisis or challenge emerges, take a few minutes to answer two simple questions:

1. What is the worst outcome of this situation?
2. What should I do if the worst outcome happens?

Once you've answered these questions, you're prepared for the worst. Because things seldom turn out as badly as we can project, dealing with the crisis will likely be easier.

4

Set Clear, Realistic Goals

Self-imposed demands or unrealistic expectations are the seeds of a stressful life. Eliminating self-imposed stress is often no more than setting realistic goals.

Realistic goals are not "easy" goals. On the contrary, they should bring on a healthy level of stress by forcing you to strive. If you're a good college football player, but not endowed with outstanding physical qualities and among the top ten in your league, it's not worthwhile setting out to be an NFL linebacker. But that doesn't stop you from achieving an 11 handicap in golf or a top spot on the tennis ladder.

Realistic goal setting is the difference between mental success and the lack thereof, because success is relative. One person might consider himself rich beyond imagination if he had a million dollars; the same amount would be small change to someone like Donald Trump. Managing expectations and objectives is what reducing internal stress is all about.

START WHERE YOU ARE

Think about where you are right now in life and visualize what you want to become. Whether you're a sixteen-year-old with your entire life ahead of you, a forty-five-year-old accountant bored to death, or a sixty-four-year-old with retirement staring you in the face, this is the first instant of the rest of your life. It is your starting place.

SET REALISTIC GOALS

Unrealistic goals always create internal stress. A forty-five-year-old accountant who decides that he wants to be a rocket scientist is setting unrealistic goals. He has opportunities galore to become a part of the space program in other ways, however, ranging from working for NASA itself to being employed by the myriad contractors who serve NASA. (Relocation might be required, of course, which would impose another set of milestones and objectives to be considered and evaluated to avoid new stress.)

Realistic goal setting means being completely honest with yourself when determining what you can objectively expect. If you're a sixteen-year-old who wants to become a basketball star and you're a good but not excellent athlete, you're setting yourself up for the stress that comes from disappointment. At the same time, a good student athlete can enter an excellent university and find an exciting course of study and a career related to her interest, possibly in sports medicine or sports journalism.

A good exercise is to write down in a single sentence the "bare bones" of what you want from life. I'll give you an example: Say that you're a parent, and your goal is to raise your child as well as possible. You'd write, "I want my child to be honest and moral and have integrity and as many options as possible." From that simple sentence you can evaluate many goals, both for you and for your child. It means you have to set an example of honesty, integrity, and strong moral character. It means you have to provide your child with options, meaning education: the basics, such as the three Rs, and skills that she can always use, such as craft work, sports that reflect her physical capacities, and so on. And it means you should encourage your child to set appropriate goals for herself, as well.

VISUALIZE A PLAN

The first step in planning is to take stock of your abilities. A forty-five-year-old accountant with a good job must have developed some excellent skills and personal traits: sticking to procedure, juggling checks and balances, accuracy, reliability, setting emotions aside, and so on. There are bound to be many, and your first task is to write them down.

The second step is to identify your passions. What do you really feel strongly about? Is it model making, teaching, being in charge, your love of numbers, people, avoiding people, computers, or perhaps a sport? It can be one thing or many things. Write them down.

Third, try to match your skills and qualifications with your passions. For example, if you love teaching, can you realistically move into the teaching of accounting? If not, why not? There are lots of teaching environments; for example, most communities have adult education classes; colleges have extension programs; there are trade schools; or you could start your own tutoring program.

Once you've identified a way to match your skills and qualities to an objective, you can reduce your overall plan to realistic, tactical steps. For example, propose to the people in charge of community education in your area that an accounting course for the next session would meet community needs, perhaps a class on how to determine family cash flow and eliminate waste.

If you can take these steps, you can take control of your life.

KEEP REALISTIC EXPECTATIONS

It's important to keep realistic expectations of what things will be like once you attain your goal. For example, lawyers are among the most "career-disturbed" professionals in America. It is easy to understand why. They have set the realistic goal of becoming lawyers and have obtained that goal. Their expectations, however, are often unrealistic. Many have grown up watching lawyer shows on television in which the brilliant lawyer saves the wrongly accused underdog, or traps the killer. That is far from what the average lawyer does. In reality, it is a rare lawyer who is lucky enough to land a job with a law firm that isn't mostly real estate closings and writing wills, reading countless reports searching for minor faults, or, at best, spending countless hours in a law library searching out precedents; and that is at the pinnacle of the profession in the top law firms.

The result is that an army of people are unhappy in what they are doing. Their unhappiness results in internal stress, because they expected a career that doesn't exist. Realistic expectations are essential.

PRACTICE SELF-DISCIPLINE

After a piano concert had ended, the concert hall steward heard someone playing the piano on stage and checked to see if an unauthorized person had sneaked into the hall. Imagine his surprise to find the concert pianist, now late for the cocktail party honoring him, playing part of the concert he had just given to an enthusiastic audience. When the steward asked why, the pianist's answer was simple: "During the third movement, I realized I could play this section a little better." That's self-discipline!

The discipline shown by the pianist is the difference between very good and great. Most people who want to do well in their profession, hobby, or sport must develop the discipline necessary to achieve their potential. And that potential can be fantastic: examples include a deaf Miss America, one-legged skiers and mountain climbers, and a blind person who sailed solo from California to Hawaii. Every day we hear about people who achieve greatness. Invariably, they have three things going for them: first, talent and basic intelligence; second, parents, guardians, or mentors who encouraged and worked with them; and third, the self-discipline to keep working toward their goals long after average folks would have stopped.

SET A TIMETABLE FOR SUCCESS

It might seem that setting a schedule for yourself would increase your stress by pressuring you toward a deadline. Goal setting, discipline, planning, and hard work are all ingredients for success, however—and so is a realistic timetable. If you're a fresh graduate with a business administration degree from a good college and working in a large bank, don't set your sights on becoming the chief loan officer in two or three years. Getting to the top of your career, developing a new skill, or any other worthwhile accomplishment takes years of experience. You're facing frustration and internal stress if you aren't realistic about what you can accomplish and when.

5

Improve Your Communication with Others

Most stress related to interpersonal relationships is due to poor or inadequate communication. Take time during the day to talk with people and learn more about them, how they think, and why they act as they do. By understanding them, you have neutralized their potential to bring stress into your life.

COMPLIMENT OTHERS

Few people ever get complimented for who they are or what they've done. Sure, you get a raise and other benefits at work, but that is not quite like a round of applause or a compliment. Paying compliments is simple to do and it will pay enormous dividends in the world around you.

Resolve that you will find something good to say about every person you must deal with. For instance, "I like your tie;" "You have a nice smile;" "That was a great job you did;" "You have a beautiful family;" "Your report was really clear." It doesn't take much and you may have to search pretty hard in some cases, but do it! You can still give compliments even if you have to discuss something negative.

FIND THE POSITIVE

A boss who couldn't give his employees an annual raise couched the news by stating, "Take a moment of silence to thank your individual God that we all have a job." Then, he led into the economics that meant "no raise this year."

In the direst situations, we search for a positive anchor. When someone dies after suffering from a disease, we often say, "At least she's not in any more pain," or if someone had a massive heart attack, "It was over so quickly that he didn't suffer."

If you make a habit of searching everything for at least one positive point and sharing that point with those around you, you will find that you'll have less stress. The stressors are still there, but your mental outlook has been elevated so they don't seem quite as overwhelming. You've made yourself taller instead of pulling the world down to your height.

ASK QUESTIONS

Inside each grown person is a child who wants to be heard. Most people like to talk about themselves and get recognition for what they've done, who they are, and what they think. So ask them!

A simple door opener is to compliment someone with a question; for example,

- "Your reports are always so clear. Did you study journalism?" or "Your questions always bring out the important technical issues. Did you study science?" That is bound to start a discussion of education, or at least the person's ability to write clearly.

- "I love the emphasis you put on words. Is that a Midwestern accent I detect?" Before you know it, you'll be discussing where that person is from, always a great topic of conversation. After all, everyone is from somewhere.

LISTEN

Most people have something to say, so listen to them. Ask a question and then let them talk. You can coach them along with little things such as, "How fascinating," or "How difficult that must have been," or "What did you do then?" Usually you'll learn information that will help you work and play with people more productively.

6

Change Type A to Type B Behavior

In the 1950s, *Type A Behavior and Your Heart* by Dr. Meyer Friedman was published. Research done by Dr. Friedman and many other scientists established that heart disease, especially heart attacks and stroke, was stress related. It was not necessarily the stress imposed on people that was making them sick, however; it was the stress they were imposing on themselves.

Research proved that people could be divided into two personality types, A or B. The Type A personalities had much higher rates of heart disease, heart attacks, and strokes than the Type B personalities. Not all the Type As had heart attacks, of course, nor did all the Type Bs avoid them. In addition, Type A people seemed to be "ulcer carriers"—they didn't seem to ever get them, yet Type B people did. Once the research was finished, however, it was clear that there are other prices that Type A people pay for their behavior.

TYPE A BEHAVIOR

If you're a Type A personality, your life is characterized by high discharges of adrenaline and cortisol. You are likely to also have high levels of cholesterol, blood fat, and blood pressure, and even to have high blood levels of clotting chemicals. These risks increase as you age, so the sooner you do something about them, the better chance you have of neutralizing them.

This personality type is very competitive. Type As have a very hard time listening and preventing themselves from taking control in conversations. In many cases they never have enough money, a large enough home, enough friends, or enough of anything else for that matter, because they subconsciously and consciously relate everything to their ability to accomplish things.

Type As cannot relax. A vacation with idle time stresses them because they interpret it as time with nothing to do. At social gatherings, they will not only turn a conversation around to the topic they want, they will dominate it as well; or they will eavesdrop, slowly inject themselves into a conversation, and then take it over.

TYPE B BEHAVIOR

Type Bs are the opposite of all of the above. They enjoy recreation and can have fun doing nothing. They are not all wrapped up in their accomplishments and often don't mention them unless asked. They seldom become angry or irritable. Relaxing or pursuing a hobby does not make them feel guilty.

CHANGING TYPE A BEHAVIOR TO TYPE B BEHAVIOR

If you recognize yourself in the description of Type As, use the following chart to compare what you have to lose to what you have to gain by changing your behavior.

Benefits of Changing Type A to Type B Behavior

Change from . . .	Change to . . .
Driving against deadlines, which are often set unnecessarily aggressively by an internal clock.	Setting realistic deadlines that are appropriately competitive.
Impatience with everything, especially with people, including family, friends, and colleagues.	Being patient with people, promoting a healthy balance at work, with family, and with friends and colleagues.
Being defined by work, because it represents the number one interest.	Balancing work, family, and recreation.
Having to come in first, dominate the conversation, be the authority.	Being confidently competitive to complete projects on an agreed-on, realistic timetable.
Being forceful in speech, actions, and human relations.	Being comfortable in conversation; learning from others.
Never listening, only waiting to talk.	Being persuasive in speech, and confident and deliberate in actions; listening carefully and speaking clearly when you can contribute or are asked.

If that is not enough to convince you, think of what it will do for your health. You will:

- Avoid high cholesterol and the need for cholesterol-lowering drugs in the future.
- Avoid high triglycerides.
- Avoid high blood pressure and the drugs to lower it, with all their side effects.
- Avoid high blood sugar.
- Avoid high levels of blood-clotting factors.

About 70 percent of personality is genetic. That genetic base is shaped, changed, and honed by our parental nurturing, peer group, and the practical need to get ahead and earn a living. If you can overcome half that inherited part (35 percent) and change the remaining 30 percent, you can convert about 65 percent of Type A behavior to Type B. This is a pretty healthy blend that should allow you to succeed, as well as live long enough to enjoy your success.

How to Change

Simply deciding to go from Type A (or A–) to perhaps Type B+ is only the first step, but it is an important decision you won't regret. Making the change requires focusing on two behavior patterns from which most of the others follow: first, time urgency, and second, aggressive competitiveness. In Type As these patterns are so strong as to be compulsive.

Time urgency manifests as different characteristics: finishing other people's sentences when you're having a conversation; feeling fidgety when waiting, even when there is nothing you or anyone else can do to speed up the process; arriving early to meetings, for flights, and so forth; speedy driving, wanting to "make time"; and an inability to enjoy unstructured, noncompetitive relaxation. Decreasing time urgency means managing your time more effectively and working more efficiently. Reread chapter 3 on priorities, and reset yours. Set priorities by the week or even by the month, and use those to determine your daily priorities. Use a calendar rather than a stopwatch.

It is important for Type As to have a daily "to do" list derived from the week's priorities. Set time aside each day for the unexpected. If the unexpected doesn't occur, use that time for meditation or other stress-relieving techniques described in upcoming chapters. Don't use the time to get ahead on other projects unless they're really important for concrete reasons, not just those in your own mind.

Screen the outside world. Put the answering machine to work. If you've got a task scheduled and do not want to be disturbed, hang a sign that politely and diplomatically says, "Go away." Stick to your guns and people will eventually get the message. After all, you'll have to train people to treat you as a Type B; they've known you only as a Type A.

Type A behavior is almost always triggered in uncontrollable situations. When such situations occur, look carefully at your priorities, assess your options in writing if possible, and compare them against your goals. You can't control the uncontrollable, but you can control the way you respond. It will be tough at first, but it will slowly become your habit.

Consider three points:

1. Can anything fail because it was done too well or too slowly?
2. Should you decide when your workday will be finished before it starts?
3. Should you keep working on your project at "quitting time"?

Each question can be answered no.

The second Type A behavior you'll need to change is aggressive competitiveness. Type A people become hostile very quickly and instantly move into a competitive mode. (Anger management is discussed in detail in chapter 9.) When those feelings start surfacing, use them as your signal to relax. Ask yourself some pertinent questions: "Am I trying to get this person to do something against his basic needs or personality?" "Am I forcing an imaginary deadline?" "Am I becoming angry or anxious because this is not moving fast enough according to my internal deadline?"

Recognize that many people either consciously or subconsciously try to precipitate an argument. So, you must instantly decide if entering the argument has any relevance to your objectives and priorities. In short, will it bring you anything you want or need? If the answer is yes, then you need to figure out how to do it without anger. If the answer is no, shut up!

Establish Type B Behavior

We live in a Type A world, and living as a Type B takes courage. In addition, being a Type B is actually difficult for someone who is naturally a Type A personality. Once you get started, however, you'll find the change is what we call an autocatalytic process—that is, it feels so good that it drives itself along.

Now that you have decided to go from Type A to Type B behavior, approach social situations with the objectives you have established here. Use them to listen to others and expand your awareness of Type B personalities and people. You will slowly find social situations more interesting and realize there are people all around you who are incredible and fascinating and who have accomplished fantastic things.

Going from Type A to Type B is like asking people to give money to a worthy cause—most people mistakenly say, "Give 'til it hurts!" but the smart solicitor says, "Give 'til it feels good!"

Tips for Type B Behavior

- Expand your interests outside of work.
- Expand your friendships with Type B people.
- Take lunch and rest breaks.
- Appreciate things for which you never had time before.
- Revive old traditions or create new ones.
- Establish at least one hobby.
- Always say to yourself, "I deserve to enjoy that."

7

Challenge Your Own Beliefs

Feelings are not caused by events! They are caused by the beliefs we carry in our minds when the events occur.

ONE EVENT, FOUR FEELINGS

Consider the reactions of four employees after being told that their company's sales are below those expected, and therefore the company's profits—and their incomes—will decline:

- I'm in deep trouble! I borrowed against our house to buy that SUV, counting on the annual bonus to bail me out. Now, with no bonus, I'll fall behind on my payments.
- This could work to my advantage. I will submit the analysis I've been doing on the new area of potential sales, and I'll dust off and rewrite the profit improvement plan everyone ignored two years ago when everything was going well.
- Big deal. I've been through these cycles before. Okay, so I don't get a bonus for a couple of years and my retirement

fund will suffer a little. I can still make my house payments, and we don't owe any other money.

- This is the boost I've needed to dust off my résumé. I've been watching things closely and saw this coming, so I'm going to find a new job with a company that's better managed.

Only the first person is seriously stressed; the second person sees this as an opportunity to turn events to his advantage; the third person reacts with indifference; and the fourth person sees an opportunity for positive change.

- We are not disturbed by things, but by our views of them.
- Only our thoughts can make an event turn out good or bad.
- You will be as happy as you decide to be.
- You can set yourself up for disaster.

BELIEFS

The relationship between events is quite basic. Albert Ellis, the famous psychologist, made it as simple as ABC:

Activating events
Beliefs we carry when the event occurs
Consequences, the emotional responses

Suppose your spouse leaves you a message saying you've got to prepare dinner for yourself this evening, as she will be working late. You could have various reactions: anger, because you feel it's your spouse's responsibility to make dinner; pride, because your spouse believes you are really quite capable of preparing a nice dinner; or fear, because you think your spouse is losing interest in your relationship and is meeting someone else on the side.

Each reaction exposes one of your inner beliefs. If your beliefs are causing you stress—internally, in your personal relationships, and so on—you've got to change them!

EXPOSING AND CHANGING YOUR INNER BELIEFS

Put your beliefs outside yourself. Review some past situations in which you were clobbered and try to determine why you reacted as you did. A good exercise is to remove the situation from your mind and put it on paper. Use the ABC concept, and follow these steps:

1. Expose Your Beliefs

   • Identify the activating event: for example, you were called to your boss's office; someone tells you your clothes don't match; or you were wrong about something.
   • Identify the belief you brought to the situation: I'm being reprimanded; I'm unsure of my clothing selection; I must always be right.
   • Identify the consequences of your belief: stress before you're even told why you were called to the office; anger that you didn't dress correctly; anxiety that you made a mistake.

Once you've reviewed your beliefs, step up to the plate and take positive action.

2. Take Positive Action

   • Dispute your belief: the boss could be wrong; my clothes are clean and well pressed—if the color's off, I'll simply coordinate better; no one can always be right.
   • Try to adopt a less stressful response: What could have gone wrong? How do I explain it? What responsibility is mine? I'll get a book or lesson on clothing coordination so it won't happen again; let's review it again so I'll see where my process was off the mark.

8

Eliminate Anxiety

Anxiety comes from negative thoughts hatched within our minds. These negative thought patterns usually date back to what our parents said to or about us and have slowly progressed through our lives, becoming the things we tell ourselves.

LESSONS LEARNED IN CHILDHOOD

When parents say things to or about their children, the children receive two messages: one is external and one is subconscious.

Suppose a child is told to put away his toys, and thirty minutes later his mother finds him doing something else and the toys untouched. She gets angry and says, "Why are you so lazy?" or "Why do you disobey me?"

No matter what the child answers, even if he jumps up immediately and proceeds to clean up the toys, his mind receives messages: I'm lazy, or I'm disobedient. If that child gets those messages often enough, he will eventually do as he is told by becoming lazy or disobedient.

Now think about people around you and try and conjure up some messages they received as children:

- Someone who is always late
- Someone who always argues with you
- Someone who speaks only when asked a direct question
- Someone whose clothes are always unkempt
- Someone who can't look you in the eye
- Someone who always backs down in an argument

What messages do you think these people were given in childhood? Did they ever overcome those messages? Is the adult still carrying and acting out those messages? If these messages aren't neutralized by more positive messages, will his success and interpersonal relations continue to be limited by them?

Negative messages provoke anxiety throughout life, and we must exchange them for positive, more realistic messages. We have to learn to ask why and then move on with some optimism.

SELF-TALK

Controlling anxiety calls for talk—self-talk. Yes, you do talk to yourself, even have discussions with yourself. Ideally, those discussions get to the root of a problem. Don't stand in crowded places having discussions with yourself out loud, but do it silently, preferably alone in a quiet place.

Start by asking yourself questions. As we saw in the last chapter, positive questions are always effective in keeping any conversation going, with yourself as well as with others. Here are some examples:

- Why have things turned out like this?
- What did I do to make it this way?
- What can I do to make the situation better? For me? For others?
- When will it become better if I take action now?
- How can I prevent this from happening in the future?

Do's and Don'ts

When you feel anxiety mounting, turn negative thoughts into positive thoughts. The best thoughts are those that don't use indefinites, such as "should have" and "would have" and those that don't tell you *not* to feel something, such as "Don't get scared" when you *are* scared. Continually try to find words with a more positive meaning. You'll find you never have problems, only challenges.

When you enter a stressful situation and anxiety starts to build, send only positive messages to your brain to cancel out any negative ones that lurk there.

Do say to yourself . . .
- What do I have to do?
- I chose to be here.
- I won't do anything out of fear!
- There are several ways to handle this.
- I am (or will be) organized and effective.
- I have emerged successful in similar situations.
- I'll pause, take some deep breaths, and gather my thoughts.

Don't say to yourself . . .
- There is too much to do.
- I have to do this.
- This is frightening.
- I think (or hope) I can handle this.
- I can't forget what I need to do.
- I'll try not to worry about the outcome.
- They say deep breathing lessens anxiety.

When you're already in the stressful situation, other positive self-talk phrases can help.

Do say to yourself . . .

- Time to relax even more.
- I can meet this challenge.
- I'll take it one step at a time.
- I'll think through this.
- I'm in control.

Don't say to yourself . . .

- I feel myself tensing up; time to relax.
- I think (or hope) I'll be all right.
- I can't handle it.
- I'll just do what I have to do.
- Don't get nervous now.

When the stressful situation continues and you're right in the thick of things, and all your childhood monsters, failures, and self-doubts are starting to build, send them running.

Do say to yourself . . .

- Okay, I feel a little nervous; that's good. I'm also confident.
- Do what I fear and the fear dies!
- I'll pause here and reassess.
- A little fear is a good motivation to bring out my best.
- I just have to manage fear, not eliminate it.

Don't say to yourself . . .

- Don't get nervous and blow this.
- Don't get scared now.
- Don't slow down now.
- Don't be afraid.
- Don't let anxiety show.
- I have to stop being scared.

Once the stressful situation is over, review your actions. You'll carry your thoughts about what has happened into the next stressful situation you encounter.

Do say to yourself . . .

- I tried hard and I got much of what I wanted.
- That could have been a complete disaster. I saved the day.
- I succeeded in several ways; next time I'll do even better.
- I did right by myself. The other person (people) can take a lesson from that.
- Next time it will be easier.
- I'm getting better every time.

Don't say to yourself . . .

- I should have done better.
- What a disaster.
- Maybe next time.
- I hope I didn't hurt their feelings.
- I hope it is easier next time.
- I'm not doing as well as I should.

9

Make Anger Work for You

Anger is probably the most self-destructive of all emotions and is the cause of severe stress. Once anger takes over, watch out! Anger is harmful and causes job loss, relationship problems, personal injury, property loss, and even death. Preventing and controlling anger is more than important; it is absolutely essential.

Everyone has either been angry or encountered someone who is angry. Some people learn at an early age not to let their own anger take over and not to let an angry person get them upset. However, most of us have to learn by experience that when anger takes over, all sorts of bad things happen. Anger management is essential to life in the modern world. It doesn't mean you need to back down, nor does it mean you put up your fists and fight; management means you assert yourself, diffuse the anger, and settle on what is right.

PREVENTING ANGER BY CONTROLLING NEGATIVE THOUGHTS

People looking for jobs will tell you the heaviest thing in the world is the telephone when you must use it to call potential employers. It is heavy because a job seeker usually projects negative thoughts onto the person she's about to call. Instead of asking herself, "What must I do in this situation?" she'll say things such as, "She probably won't take my call," or "He'll say they don't have any openings," and so on. Negative thoughts lay the groundwork for anger if the person with whom you are interacting shows even the slightest tendency to fulfill your negative projection.

A better approach is to prepare for the worst. Write it down if it helps. For instance, "What must I do if . . ."

- He won't take my call.
- She says they have no openings now.
- He says I'm overqualified (or underqualified).
- She says, "Send me a résumé."

If you are prepared, you cannot get angry; you can only say, "I did my best; I'll do better next time."

When You Are Accused

Being blamed or accused is pretty much the equivalent of a boxing match. In the boxing ring, the announcer makes it very clear that two people are going to try and knock each other senseless.

When you are accused in workplace or personal situations, however, you'll be on the employment line, or in jail, or both rather quickly if you start throwing punches. At the same time, you must assert yourself.

Using the following phrases can help bring about fair resolution to confrontations such as these:

- Let's take this point by point.
- Perhaps we're both right. Let's take a cooperative approach.
- Arguments only lead to more arguments. Let's work together constructively.

Make sure that your statements are not accusatory, even if you feel deep inside you'd like to accuse your adversary. As you feel your anger grow, you've got to gain control of your thoughts. Try some positive self-talk, such as:

- I'll slow down here and take a few deep breaths.
- This anger is okay because it is nature's way of telling me what I must do.

If the situation doesn't require an instant solution and anger is rising, you might propose a break. This could be the right time to take a breather and return to discuss the issues, one by one, at a later time.

DAMAGE-LIMITING OPERATIONS

Think of being cut off on the road while driving. The best thing to do is pull off the road, collect your thoughts, give the bad driver a chance to get far away, and resolve to drive more defensively. Most anger-producing effects, however, are not so final as being cut off. Suppose you've been sold a defective product or been cheated. Your objective is to stop the loss, recover what you can, move on, and avoid similar losses in the future. The techniques you use are called damage-limiting operations, because you've already lost something and you want to prevent future losses, or limit the damage that's been done.

Anger is positive in such cases. Thank your body for alerting you to the seriousness of the problem, and get back in control of the situation by focusing on the future and limiting the damage.

For example, suppose you were accused (even jokingly) out loud at a party of hitting your spouse. Some people will always be ready to believe the worst. For the sake of your relationships and reputation, you've got to find a way to convince as many people as possible that you don't hit your loved ones.

Several approaches immediately spring to mind, such as slugging your accuser and shouting, "It's a lie!" but these actions won't convince many people; in fact, observers will only be more likely to believe the accusation.

Instead, you might try putting one of these questions to your accuser:

- Why would you joke about something so serious?
- Whoever told you that?
- Should I dignify that insult, or will you admit you're joking?
- Who put you up to saying that?

Notice that your reply is built around your own confidence that the truth is with you. You are not defensive, nor are you directly accusing your adversary of lying. And by implying it is a joke, you are offering him a way out of the dilemma he has created for himself.

HANDLING ANGER DURING STRESSFUL SITUATIONS

When you are entering a stressful situation that is almost sure to cause anger, your objective is to prevent that anger.

Do say to yourself . . .
- What do I have to do?
- How many ways are there to deal with this?
- There may not be a need to argue.
- I'll take three deep breaths, collect my thoughts, and relax.
- A sense of humor will be very helpful.

Don't say to yourself . . .
- I have to win.
- I'm going to get angry.
- There is going to be an argument.
- I'm ready for him (her, them).
- I'm serious.

If you're in a situation where your anger is building and you can't leave, you've got to see it through—but try to control your anger.

Do say to yourself . . .

- I'm starting to get tense; time to slow down.
- Anger's a good signal; now it's time to control and help myself.
- Let's take this one point at a time.
- Could we both be right?
- Could a cooperative effort work?
- Let's focus on what is right here.
- Let's work together constructively.
- I'm not going to get angry.

Don't say to yourself . . .

- I'm all tensed up.
- This makes me mad.
- He is wrong.
- They are against me.
- She started this argument.
- I'll show him.

If the situation has become very tense, make use of some damage-limiting techniques.

Do say to yourself . . .

- I'll keep my cool and will be in control.
- What do I want to get out of this?
- I do not need to prove myself.
- I'll try and contain this.
- What he says may not matter at all.
- There have to be some good parts to this. What are they?

Don't say to yourself . . .

- He can't do that.
- I'll get even.
- I won't let him get away with that.
- I'll take it right to the top.
- He can't say that to me.
- This will be awful.

After the situation is resolved, no matter how it turned out, go to a quiet place and assess what you've been through.

Do say to yourself . . .

- These difficult situations take time to work out.
- I resolve to try and not take it personally.
- That could have been worse; or, it wasn't as tough as I thought.
- I'm making progress!

Don't say to yourself . . .

- "Stuff" happens.
- He never did see my point.
- That was awful.
- I should have said more.
- I'll win next time.

10

Avoid High Blood Pressure

High blood pressure is both the most prevalent and the most preventable disease among adults. Its prevalence among adults is the best indicator of how high the stress level has becoming in our modern, competitive society. Worse, high blood pressure is becoming a problem for the teenage population, which means that it will only be more prevalent in the future.

HYPERTENSION: THE SILENT KILLER

High blood pressure, or hypertension, is called the "silent killer" because its symptoms are so mild and usually develop so slowly that most people don't know they have it until a doctor tells them. The symptoms of hypertension are summarized in the following chart.

People with hypertension seldom experience all these symptoms, and many never have any. In addition, symptoms can be so mild or start so slowly that a person becomes accustomed to them. After all, who hasn't had a headache or a nosebleed? Been dizzy? Felt depressed? This is what makes hypertension such an insidious disease.

Common Symptoms of Hypertension	
• Morning headaches	• Blurred vision
• Ringing in the ears	• Tension when there's no cause
• Unexplained dizziness	• Flushing or redness of the face
• Spontaneous nosebleeds	and nose
• Depression without apparent cause	• Fainting spells

WHAT IS BLOOD PRESSURE?

Blood pressure is expressed as the relationship between two types of pressure: systolic and diastolic. Systolic pressure is the pressure exerted when your heart beats and forces the blood through the arteries. Diastolic pressure is the pressure between heartbeats. We express blood pressure as the ratio of these two numbers, with systolic over diastolic. Both numbers are expressed in millimeters of mercury, and systolic pressure should be about forty millimeters higher than diastolic pressure. For example, my blood pressure is usually 105 systolic and 65 diastolic. I would write it simply as 105/65 or say it as "one-oh-five over sixty-five."

Blood pressure is measured with a sphygmomanometer, a big word for a simple device. It consists of three parts: the cuff, a device to detect sound, and a pressure sensor. The cuff goes around your arm and is pumped full of air so it stops the blood flow. The cuff is hooked to a column of mercury or a pressure sensor that shows the pressure inside the cuff. The nurse puts a stethoscope or other listening device just below the cuff to listen for specific sounds, known as the Korotkoff sounds. The nurse slowly releases the cuff pressure and listens. At first, because the cuff is tight, she hears nothing. Then she slowly releases the cuff pressure and hears *thump-thump-*

thump. This thumping is the heart pushing blood past the cuff with each beat, and the pressure at this point is the systolic pressure. Cuff pressure is allowed to fall just until these thumps are replaced by a steady whooshing sound. Pressure at the instant the whoosh appears is the diastolic pressure.

You can purchase a device that measures blood pressure electronically. Electronic sphygmomanometers are available in drugstores and by mail order. They usually have a cuff that fits on the arm, which contains a sensitive listening device, so you only need to pump up the cuff and the instrument does the rest. In fact, some of them even pump up the cuff for you! Others use your thumb to take the measurements, and some have a digital readout of systolic pressure, diastolic pressure, and pulse rate.

WHAT'S NORMAL? WHAT'S HIGH?

When diastolic blood pressure reaches 85 millimeters, I think it is too high. When systolic pressure reaches 150, with diastolic below 90, it is too high. As with most other serious health issues, the surgeon general has set standards, summarized in Table 10.1.

High blood pressure is called hypertension, so someone with hypertension is a hypertensive person. As a practical matter, when diastolic blood pressure reaches 85 regularly, it is time to take action. A person with blood pressure at that level has a 10 percent greater risk of an early death than someone whose blood pressure is lower.

HIGH BLOOD PRESSURE IS AN ENVIRONMENTAL DISEASE

High blood pressure usually creeps up slowly, so to assign a single cause other than heredity (which accounts for about 2 to 3 percent of all cases of high blood pressure) cannot be done. Calling high

---

Table 10.1

Classification of High Blood Pressure
(range in millimeters of mercury)

Diastolic Blood Pressure	Category of High Blood Pressure
Less than 85	Normal
85 to 89	High normal
90 to 104	Mild hypertension
105 to 114	Moderate hypertension
115 or higher	Severe hypertension

Systolic Blood Pressure with Diastolic Blood Pressure Less Than 90	
Less than 140	Normal
140 to 159	Borderline Isolated Systolic Hypertension
160 or more	Isolated Systolic Hypertension

---

blood pressure an environmental disease is a polite way of saying it has many causes.

Type A Behavior

People who are very tense and live a life of internally generated stress generally develop high blood pressure. Type A behavior might be good for getting ahead in business, but it is detrimental to living a longer life. See chapter 6 for tips on reducing Type A behavior.

External Stress

Stress is often a factor in the workplace, but it can also exist in the home, in the neighborhood, and among friends. If you can't eliminate external stress or take steps to reduce its impact, you will likely develop high blood pressure. It is a symptom that something is awry in your life.

Smoking

Smoking can cause high blood pressure all by itself. Two toxic chemicals from cigarette smoke constrict the arteries and capillaries and interfere with metabolism. Smoking is a habit people often take up as a result of external stress. (For more on smoking and stress, see chapter 11.)

Alcohol

Excessive alcohol intake always causes high blood pressure in people who are particularly sensitive to alcohol, and it makes high blood pressure worse for everyone. Alcohol-related high blood pressure usually doesn't respond to blood pressure medication; it's the alcohol intake itself that has to be stopped. (For more on stress and alcohol, see chapter 22.)

Excess Weight

Being overweight causes high blood pressure for two reasons: first, each pound of fat requires about five miles of small blood vessels called capillaries, and the heart must use higher pressure to push the blood through those many extra miles. Second, overweight people produce an excess of the hormone insulin. Excess insulin causes the kidneys to raise blood pressure.

Overweight people who have high blood pressure must lose weight and straighten out a few other dietary factors, such as adopting a low-sugar, high-carbohydrate diet with a balanced K-factor (the ratio of sodium to potassium in the diet); when they do so, their high blood pressure usually disappears completely. (For tips on losing excess weight, see chapter 16.)

Poor Dietary Habits

Too much salt in the diet is the basis of much high blood pressure. Salt upsets the K-factor (chapter 17 is devoted to the management of K-factor). Many other dietary elements contribute to high blood pressure by causing constant recurring stress:

- *Fiber:* only 5 percent of adults get adequate dietary fiber.
- *Calcium and magnesium:* these are a basis for sensible supplements.
- *Fat balance:* imbalance is caused by excessive saturated fat and insufficient omega-3 oils.

Fitness

Sedentary people have an unfit vascular system; regular exercise will reduce blood pressure all by itself. Regular exercise develops more flexibility in blood vessels so when the heart beats, blood is forced not into a rigid set of pipes but into an elastic and yielding system. Hence, less pressure is required to get the blood where it is going. It's as if the arteries help the blood along rather than resist its flow.

MEASURE YOUR PULSE

Learn to measure your pulse. It is an easy indicator of your stress level and is excellent for relaxation and biofeedback techniques.

1. Begin by sitting, with the elbow of your right arm resting on a midchest-high support. A table or desk is usually convenient.
2. Find your pulse on the underside of your right wrist. It is on the outside as you look down while holding your palm up.
3. Use the first three fingers of your left hand to find the pulse on your right wrist.
4. Once you find your pulse, count it for a full minute.

Experiment with your pulse. Take it after you run upstairs, when you are nervous or relaxed, during and after exercise, when you are stressed out, and at other times. When you are seated and relaxed, your pulse should be about 70 to 75 beats per minute or less. A lower resting heart rate usually characterizes a healthy cardiovascular system. For example, a well-conditioned athlete usually has a resting heart rate below 50.

11

Quit Smoking (and If You Don't Smoke, Don't Start!)

Smoking is a major stress on the body. People often claim they smoke to relieve stress; in fact, smoking reduces a person's ability to cope with stress. The reason for this is very simple: Smoking reduces the amount of oxygen available for normal metabolism because the chemicals in cigarette smoke, mainly carbon monoxide, bind the oxygen, making it unavailable. Reduced oxygen means that carbohydrate metabolism can't rise to necessary levels; that is why smokers get out of breath quickly when they run.

More important, the brain relies on carbohydrate metabolism for all its energy. Therefore, when the body is under stress and the fight-or-flight response kicks in, energy for thought and activity isn't there when required. Just when you need a clear mind, you have reduced your ability to respond. It is as if a runner decided to put a pebble in one shoe just before the race—not too smart.

While I can offer some good nutritional advice to help prevent cancer and other smoking-related diseases, there is only one way to overcome this oxygen shortfall: Stop smoking!

GRIM STATISTICS

Smoking causes lung cancer and increases the risk of just about every other type of cancer. Besides that, it is a major risk factor in heart disease, stroke, ulcers, and emphysema. Smoking also affects skin tone and color and reduces physical ability, especially stamina.

Smoking causes one in six deaths and half of all strokes among people under the age of sixty-five. Lung cancer is second only to heart disease as a cause of death in women. Smoking is just about one of the worst addictive habits in the world.

Ulcers

Smoking increases the risk of ulcers. Prostaglandins, one of a unique group of chemicals our bodies produce, are essential for a healthy lining of the stomach and small intestine. Smoking reduces the production of these essential prostaglandins, a reduction that, when prolonged over a period of years, causes the lining of these vital digestive organs to lose tone and become susceptible to damage from the normal digestive process. In brief, ulcers slowly develop.

Stress is a secondary contributor to the ulcers that smokers develop. Recall that under stress the digestive process stops. This leaves the undigested stomach contents, including stomach acids, where they are. Digestive organ linings, weakened by years of smoking, are consequently more susceptible to this stress cycle, making smokers more likely than nonsmokers to get ulcers.

Heart Disease

Smokers deposit more cholesterol on their artery walls than nonsmokers. Toxic chemicals in smoke irritate the cardiac arteries. In defense, the body protects the points of irritation by applying fatty deposits. These deposits, small at first, take on a life of their own and grow, producing heart disease.

Smokers have a much greater risk of heart attack than nonsmokers, and if a smoker has a heart attack, his ability to recover is less than that of a nonsmoker. Not only does smoking compromise your health, it compromises your ability to improve your health.

Stroke

Carbon monoxide in the blood from smoking increases the clumping of certain kinds of blood cells called platelets. Clumping occurs naturally when we cut ourselves—the clump of platelets develops into a clot and the bleeding stops. When a clot forms inside a blood vessel in the head, it blocks the blood flow to a part of the brain, and that brain tissue dies. We call this a stroke.

Cosmetic Effects

Smokers develop more facial wrinkles than nonsmokers and a somewhat grayish skin color. Wrinkles reflect poor production of the protein collagen, a process that requires vitamin C. Skin color discloses its composition, which is changed by an accumulation of materials from smoke that can be best compared to the stains on smokers' teeth and fingers.

Mental and Physical Stamina

The blood's reduced capacity to carry oxygen can make smokers tire more quickly. In a smoker's blood, some oxygen-carrying iron is bound with carbon monoxide. The oxygen-carrying capacity of the blood is compromised because the red blood cells are burdened with the carbon monoxide from smoke. Consequently, smokers tire more quickly and generally have reduced physical stamina. Stamina diminishes so much that many coaches won't work with athletes who smoke or have smoked, because these athletes are unable to reach their full potential.

Mental energy and mental stamina are similarly compromised by smoking, because less oxygen is supplied to the brain as well as the muscles. Thus, a person's ability to respond mentally is compromised, and his ability to concentrate for long hours is also reduced.

Although this loss of mental ability cannot be measured as precisely as can physical activity, scientists can use the eyes as a "window" into what goes on inside our heads. Precise optical measurements, which can measure subtle differences, show that the vision of smokers is consistently reduced compared to nonsmokers. Since the retina of the eye is actually a specialized brain tissue, there is no longer any question that smoking compromises mental ability; indeed, the only debate that remains is by how much.

Periodontal Disease

Teeth and gums can create more stress than any other set of tissues in the body—not because of the pain of going through the dentistry required to get tooth and gum problems fixed, but because of the subtle effects that slowly develop from periodontal disease.

Smoking, through a series of biochemical reactions that destroy vitamin C, slowly causes problems with the fibers that attach the teeth to the gums and bone. This compromised attachment gives unwanted bacteria a foothold and gum disease slowly develops. While gum disease, once clearly recognized, can be medically treated, it has other insidious effects on the body. The bacteria involved continually release toxins that exert an ongoing stress on other organs and tissues.

SMOKING AND NUTRIENT DEFICIENCIES

Many smokers will never quit, or will quit long after they should have, even though a doctor has given them bad news about their health. Smokers also tend to eat poorly. In fact, research published in the world's best medical journals has consistently reported that smokers have the following dietary problems:

- Smokers eat excessive amounts of meat.
- Smokers' diets fall far short in intake of vegetables and fruit.
- Smokers' diets fall short in intake of cereals and grains.
- Smokers tend to avoid cruciferous vegetables.
- Smokers tend to consume above-average amounts of alcohol and caffeine.
- Smokers' diets lack vitamins and minerals.

While these findings indicate that smokers have worse-than-average health, the effects of smoking don't stop there. Smokers' children, especially adolescent children, tend to have the same dietary shortfalls as their smoking parents. So, if you smoke and think it affects only you, you're sadly mistaken; it affects everyone around you. Until you quit smoking, follow the dietary recommendations given below.

Vitamin C

Smokers need at least twice the amount of vitamin C as nonsmokers; at the very least, 120 milligrams or more daily. Eat more fruits and vegetables, eat a second orange, or drink another glass of orange juice. Vitamin C supplements are also helpful.

A smoker should take a 500-milligram vitamin C supplement in the morning and in the evening, for a daily total of 1,000 milligrams.

Beta-Carotene

A smoker should eat at least two medium-size carrots daily, or about six to eight of those small, packaged carrots, which are excellent snacks. Alternatives or possible additions are half a melon or a serving of broccoli, cauliflower, brussels sprouts, or other deeply colored vegetables. Beta-carotene is a major defensive nutrient and also helps skin tone and color.

Many studies of smokers indicate that increased blood levels of beta-carotene from such natural sources have a protective effect against cancer in smokers. Beta-carotene also protects against other stresses associated with smoking. (Beta-carotene taken as a supplement does not have the same protective effects.)

Vitamin E and Selenium

Research indicates that consuming more vitamin E and selenium provides extra protection. Foods that provide beta-carotene also contain vitamin E. Add extra fruit and seafood to your diet, as well as nuts for selenium.

If you take vitamin E and selenium in supplement form, don't take more than 150 micrograms of selenium daily. The amount of vitamin E isn't a problem up to about 3,000 milligrams daily, which is the limit researchers have used.

12

Neutralize the Effects of Carbon Monoxide and Air Pollution

You may have skipped the last chapter because you're not a smoker. However, there is a good chance you already smoke and don't know that you do. People who commute by car and sit in traffic jams at intersections and bridges smoke. They don't necessarily use cigarettes or pipes, but carbon monoxide levels in their blood match those of people who smoke from one-half to one pack of cigarettes daily; people who commute by bus or use other poorly ventilated public transportation methods face the same problem.

Although the evidence is not as compelling for people who spend a lot of time in airports or on crowded airplanes, they too are breathing foul air. This increases the need for the antioxidant vitamins C and E and for the other antioxidants described in this chapter.

FREE RADICALS

People who can't avoid commuting can still neutralize the stress this "secondhand smoking" imposes on their bodies, the effects of which can be summarized in one sentence: Foul air creates free radicals and includes many toxic chemicals.

Free radicals are oxidizing agents, similar in a way to a lit match. The difference is they don't give off light, last for only an instant, and work at a level so microscopic they can't be seen. The results, on an ultramicroscopic level, however, are almost the same—tissue is damaged, just as if it were burned.

The transient chemical structure of free radicals involves an unpaired electron. This unpaired electron is "loose" and looking for attachment at any cost. We say a free radical is highly reactive, because nature must combine it with something very quickly to maintain harmony. If the free radical combines with an important material, it can do irreparable, even deadly, damage. Think of free radicals as superexplosives that can destroy small, essential parts of a living system. These reactions take place at the molecular level, so we can't even watch them with the most powerful microscope. All we can do is assess the accumulated damage of myriad reactions later on when they show up as a health defect, such as heart disease, cancer, cataracts, or emphysema.

When a free radical interacts with something in our blood or any body fluid, it can produce a foreign material that may be a toxin. If a cancer-causing toxin is produced, we can expect big trouble later on; if it's a rancid oil in place of an oil our bodies need, it could gum up a natural metabolic process, sort of the way a stalled car on a bridge causes traffic to back up, even on routes other than those that lead directly to the bridge.

Once a toxin is produced, the body must get rid of it. This means passing it through the excretory system, including the kidneys, bladder, and the intestinal tract. If we continue producing the toxin, we increase the chances of overwhelming our other defenses, and our risk from the toxin's effects—for example, the chances it can cause cancer or high blood pressure—will also increase. The longer we expose ourselves to the oxidizing agent without neutralizing it or the toxins it can produce, the greater our risk.

ANTIOXIDANTS TO THE RESCUE

In over four billion years, nature has developed many ways to deal with free radicals and oxidizing agents. The antioxidant materials in plants that protect photosynthesis—that prevent ripe fruit from going bad, oils from becoming rancid, and so on—are useful to all animals, including humans, that eat them.

We are still in the process of learning about antioxidants. We know that some nutrients, such as vitamins C and E, have a dual role: They are essential in the chemical processes that make up metabolism, and also are effective as antioxidants. The recommended dietary intake (RDI for short) of many nutrients the body needs as vitamins is usually for very small amounts; the body needs much higher amounts of these nutrients for them to be effective as antioxidants.

Drugstores, health food stores, and grocery stores, as well as Internet health sites, sell many antioxidants in pill form. Outside of a very few studies on vitamins C and E and beta-carotene, there is little scientific support for the use of these various antioxidants, and some data suggest they could, under certain circumstances, be detrimental to health.

Rather than taking antioxidants in pill and capsule form, study after study shows that people who get these antioxidants from natural foods have fewer diseases and generally live longer. The reasons are very complex because natural foods, such as carrots, provide many materials in subtle ratios that we don't yet understand. Vitamin E, for instance, provides us the collective antioxidant activity of eight different components. The notion that simply putting these antioxidants in a pill is the same as getting them from the food we eat is preposterous.

SHORING UP OUR ANTIOXIDANT DEFENSES

Because antioxidants are obtained from food and food supplements, we tend to think of our bodies as passive, simply taking antioxidants from food for our defensive needs. It's not that way at all. We naturally have a very active antioxidant capacity that is strengthened by eating the correct foods:

- Eat deep green, dark red, orange, or yellow vegetables: three to five servings daily.
- Eat fruits with red, yellow, orange, or green flesh: three to five servings daily.
- If you're a coffee drinker, choose tea in place of coffee for one cup daily. If you can make a complete switch, evidence indicates tea is better than coffee.
- Drink colored fruit juices: 100% fruit juice, such as orange, cranberry, melon, papaya, and the like.
- If you don't drink hot beverages, learn to drink iced tea made from loose tea, not instant tea.

If you decide to take extra antioxidants in supplement form, do so in moderation. Serious clinical research indicates that excesses can have a detrimental effect.

Antioxidant Supplements

- *Vitamin C:* As much as 1,000 milligrams is good for someone who smokes. Make sure the supplement contains bioflavonoids.
- *Beta-carotene:* Up to 25 milligrams daily, in addition to lots of colored vegetables.
- *Vitamin E:* 100 international units (IU) up to 1,500 IU daily.

13

Meditate

Studies conducted on people before and after beginning a meditation program showed some startling effects. Once their meditation program was well established, their blood pressure dropped, their resting pulse was lower, they slept more soundly, and their cholesterol was lower.

How can that be? Think about everything you've read about stress: it causes elevated blood pressure, more rapid pulse, and elevated cholesterol, and the anxiety that stress produces steals sleep. It follows that meditation is a sort of "antistress" process.

Meditation was described by Professor Herbert Benson, M.D., of Harvard Medical School as the "relaxation response." Relaxation is a nice general definition; however, meditation as a process can fill volumes, and there are various methods of meditation practice.

There are some characteristics, however, that are basic to every method. A teacher is always preferable if you're really serious, but meditation is something you can learn on your own. A few basic principles can get anyone started.

MEDITATION BASICS

You should set aside a block of time—preferably fifteen minutes until you become proficient at reaching a meditative state—during which you can be completely alone. This is a time during which any phone in your immediate vicinity is shut off and other phones are set on the answering machine. There should be no radios or TVs on within close earshot, nor shouting or other loud noises. Early morning or late evening may be best. Find a quiet place where nobody will interrupt you during your allotted time frame. This could be a room or a forest glade, or you might even use your car. For beginners, it is best to have a room or even a large closet that is isolated. Some people start by using the attic in their home. Once you get the hang of meditation, you can do it almost any place you can scrape out ten to twenty minutes for yourself.

Teachers of meditation usually have students assume the relaxed lotus position: sit on the floor with your back relaxed, arms on your knees, which are raised somewhat, and your feet with soles facing each other about a foot apart. Alternatively, some people sit in a soft chair. If you're meditating in a forest glade, sit on the ground in the lotus position, or on a rock. In any position, your hands should be relaxed and preferably resting on your legs.

Teachers of meditation usually assign students a mantra to recite over and over. These mantras are, as a rule, more sounds than words; they become the focus of your attention. Instead, you may focus on a feeling, possibly even visualize a nice scene, such as a mountain lake where no wind can reach. Your eyes should be closed throughout this period of reflection.

Our world is filled with distractions, and meditation is sometimes assisted by what is called white noise. This is not music, but noise that becomes a background setting for your meditation. Meditation tapes of background noises such as quiet surf, a wooden sailing ship, or wind in a forest are often sold in shops and catalogues. These sounds create a background that helps you relax.

To say that's all there is to meditation would be untrue, of course. If you are interested in pursuing meditation, you can find beginning, intermediate, and advanced classes in your area.

HOW LONG SHOULD YOU MEDITATE?

Anyone who starts meditation learns quickly that two minutes can seem like two hours, or even two days. Rather than open your eyes and check a clock, set a timer that doesn't tick. An electronic, battery-operated timer can be purchased in any hardware store. Start with a five-minute setting and continue until it rings. Then increase the time until you are meditating at least fifteen minutes. Once you achieve fifteen minutes, you will begin to notice a change in your ability to deal with stress.

I recommend twenty minutes of quiet time each day. After you have meditated for about fifteen minutes and are relaxed, use that remaining time to reaffirm who you are and what you will become. This "self-talk" should affirm that you will be optimistic and positive; similarly, you should reaffirm not to allow anger, anxiety, or fear to take over your thoughts.

14

Learn to Relax

Telling an adult he must learn to relax is like telling him that he must learn to breathe. Very few people, however, really know how to relax. Indeed, some people think that tense muscles are a sign of strength. They're wrong. Tense muscles are really a sign of wasted energy. Learning to relax is not learning to be lazy; on the contrary, it is learning how to use energy for important things.

Muscle groups around the head, including the face, neck, and shoulders, are generally more likely to tense up under stress. In some people, tenseness comes to the arms, hands, chest, stomach, and especially the back, which also involves the hips. In some situations— for example, when driving—the legs and feet are likely to tense up. Pay attention to which muscle groups become tense when you're under stress. When you feel them become tense in the future, you'll recognize that you're under stress and you will be better able to relax.

Just as you exercise daily to gain fitness, you need to relax progressively to become good at relaxing. The advantage of learning progressive relaxation is that it doesn't require special clothes or shoes; it can be done just about anywhere; and once you get good at it, you can employ the techniques whenever things become stressful. Then, while everyone around you is stressed out, you will be able to remain relaxed and in control.

PROGRESSIVE RELAXATION

Progressive relaxation involves tensing a muscle group to a point where the group is tight, but not to the point where it's quivering, and holding that point for a count of five. Then let go and let the muscle group relax.

An easy way to practice this technique is to tighten your arm muscle while sitting in a chair with someone holding your hand. Then, have your partner try to lift your arm while it's tensed. Assuming that your partner isn't a weight lifter trying to prove her strength, she shouldn't be able to lift it if you're tensing it correctly. Then close your eyes, let your arm relax, and see if your partner can lift your hand.

Call your fully tensed position a hundred, and your relaxed position zero. That range of tension is what you are trying to achieve with all your muscle groups. You should go from one group to another according to the following plan:

- Separately tense individual muscle groups.
- Hold the tension for five seconds.
- Relax the tension slowly, and say to yourself, "Relax and let go."
- Take a deep breath.
- Breathe out slowly, silently saying, "Relax and let go."

Points to Remember

- Don't tighten muscles to the point where they either hurt or become stiff.
- Understand what your muscles feel like when tensed; to some degree, that is how they will feel when you're under stress.
- Relax one muscle group at a time.

At first you should practice in a lounge chair with a footrest; this will help you isolate muscle groups and make learning easier. As you get better, you'll find you are able to do progressive relaxation almost anywhere, and it won't require as much time. Some people learn to do it during their daily commute; others do it at work during the day or at home. Whenever and wherever you can is the right time and place.

Relaxing Muscle Groups

Tense each muscle group, then relax.

Head

- Wrinkle your forehead.
- Squint your eyes tightly.
- Open your mouth wide.
- Clench your jaw tightly.
- Push your tongue to the roof of your mouth.

Neck

- Push your head back into a pillow or headrest.
- Bring your head down so your chin touches your chest.
- Roll your head to your left shoulder.
- Roll your head to your right shoulder.

Shoulders

- Shrug both shoulders as if to touch your ears.
- Shrug your right shoulder alone.
- Shrug left shoulder alone.

Arms and Hands

- Hold both arms in front of you, make fists, and tighten your arms.

- One arm at a time: push your hand against the surface on which you're resting.
- One arm at a time: from a straight position, make a fist and slowly bend your elbow, pulling your fist toward you while tightening your arm.

Chest and Lungs

- Take a deep breath; while holding, tighten your chest muscles.

Back

- Arch your back. Ideally, while lying on your stomach with your hands on the small of your back, arch your back so your head and feet are off the floor.

Stomach

- Tighten your stomach area.
- Push your stomach area out.
- Pull your stomach area in.

Hips to Feet

- Tighten your hips.
- Push your heels against the floor or footrest.
- Tighten your leg muscles below the knee.
- Curl your toes down (try to touch the bottom of your foot).
- Curl your toes up.

OTHER RELAXING PROGRAMS

There are many programs offered to help people relax. They range from do-it-yourself tapes to programs sponsored by hospitals and community centers. Each program works to some extent. However, if you use the progressive relaxation program described in this chapter, you can succeed quite well on your own.

15

Exercise

As we learned in the introduction to this book, exercise is controlled stress. Regular exercise not only builds the capacity of your entire cardiovascular system, it also builds your capacity to handle physical and emotional stress. Regular exercise dissipates the biochemical by-products of emotional stress, which include blood fats, sugar, and cholesterol, among others. It also burns off the hormonal by-products and "toxins" of stress. Most important, it reduces high blood pressure.

AEROBIC VERSUS ANAEROBIC EXERCISE

Aerobic means "with air"; *anaerobic* means "without air." Anaerobic exercise is actually a slight misnomer: you breathe when you do anaerobic exercise just as you do in aerobic, but you don't exercise your heart and arteries as much, even though you elevate your general metabolism.

Anaerobic exercise is usually short in duration, even if quite vigorous. Your body performs almost without the need to breathe. For example, running a 100-yard dash is vigorous exercise and leaves the runner gulping for air; it is considered anaerobic, because the energy used during the dash comes from energy-yielding substances within the body. Although it sounds strange, the runner could run the dash holding his breath (admittedly, it would be tough to do). He'd be gulping for air afterward to help his body replenish energy-yielding substances and rid itself of built-up wastes.

Weight lifting is a more typical example of anaerobic exercise. Everyone experiences anaerobic exercise when running up a flight of stairs or chasing a bus. The oxygen debt leaves them gulping for air.

In contrast, aerobic exercise is done for longer periods, generally longer than fifteen minutes. It requires steady breathing rather than the gulping for air that follows anaerobic exercise. Walking briskly for forty to sixty minutes, jogging for fifteen or more minutes, or swimming are all examples of aerobic exercise that require regular breathing; when finished, the person might not be out of breath even if she is sweating profusely.

Your body always needs oxygen to maintain metabolism. During aerobic exercise, metabolism is elevated for a longer period than it is during anaerobic exercise, so the body can't rely only on its high-energy reserves, or even on its carbohydrate reserves, but must burn both fat and carbohydrate—a switch that occurs about fifteen minutes into the exercise.

This metabolic shift also increases the need for oxygen, which means that your cardiovascular system must work a little harder. Essentially, you're stressing your cardiovascular system to build it up to a healthier level. Your heart and arteries—indeed, your entire cardiovascular system—are mostly muscle and require exercise more than any other system in your body. By doing some form of aerobic exercise, you prevent the buildup of fatty deposits in the arteries and even remove some. These deposits are the foundations of heart disease; preventing or eliminating them through exercise is one of the most important ways you can prevent heart disease. Exercise also prevents high blood pressure, Type 2 diabetes, and other illnesses.

Aerobic exercise works large muscle groups, such as the arms and legs, challenging the cardiovascular system. In this way, major muscle groups and the cardiovascular system are conditioned together. Aerobic fitness produces whole-body fitness. In contrast, a weight lifter can strengthen one muscle group, but might not condition his cardiovascular system, unless he also does aerobic exercise.

TRAINING EFFECT

The *training effect* is scientific jargon for having exercised and improved your cardiovascular system, as you do in aerobic exercise. You probably also have helped to build muscles, such as those in your legs and arms, in the process. When you finish, you are in better condition than when you started. Seems worth doing, doesn't it?

To get a training effect, you must:

- achieve a training heart rate quickly and do the exercise for at least twelve minutes, preferably twenty minutes; or
- achieve an increased heart rate and keep it up for at least thirty minutes, preferably one hour; or
- combine the above two requirements by achieving a modest increased heart rate and keeping it up for at least twenty minutes, preferably forty minutes.

Exercise is effective only when it is done regularly and with some rest periods, such as a day off every three or four days. You should exercise on five out of seven days. Once you have been exercising one way regularly for a year and are in shape, it is a good idea to use several different forms of aerobic exercise on different days, or weeks, to improve; each type of exercise provides its own benefits.

While exercising, the temperature inside your muscles increases to about 102 degrees Fahrenheit from its normal 98.6 degrees. That 3.4-degree rise (1 percent) increases the rate of metabolism over 17 percent, which increases circulation by at least 100 percent. This change in circulation brings more oxygen to all organs and tissues, including the brain, and, at the same time, flushes wastes (toxins) from your body. It is like a spring rain cleaning dirty streets; this is why regular exercise reduces the risk of just about every known disease.

A training heart rate is about 70 to 80 percent of the maximum rate your heart can beat safely. If you want to be precise in your exercise program, you should achieve this rate and keep it up for about twenty to thirty minutes. Table 15.1 displays average training heart rates.

Suppose you can't jog, don't have access to a pool or stair climber, or for some other reason can't exercise vigorously enough to achieve a training heart rate. Some people have no problem. A brisk forty- to sixty-minute walk will impart a training effect, even though the heart rate is below the training level. Other people can't reach a training rate easily. Some also need to exercise longer in each session. If you're one of these people, you must work a little harder to keep the gift of health you have and do even more work to make it better. And while working harder can mean running or walking faster,

Table 15.1

Training Heart Rates for Average People

Age	Maximum	75% Maximum	10-Second Pulse
20	200	150	25
25	195	146	24
30	190	143	24
35	186	140	23
40	182	140	23
45	179	134	22
50	175	131	22
55	171	128	21
60	160	120	20
Over 65	150	113	19

Table 15.2

Time Required for Exercise

Exercise	Time Required
Brisk walk	12 minutes per mile for 40 to 50 minutes
Jogging	8 minutes per mile for 25 minutes
Bicycling	25 minutes at 13 mph
NordicTrack or actual cross-country skiing	25 minutes
Leg and arm rowing machine or actually rowing in a boat with a movable seat	25 minutes
Aerobic Rider	30 minutes
Swimming laps with regular strokes	30 minutes, or 50 minutes if you are slow
Stair climber	30 minutes

doing it longer is better; you don't place as much wear and tear on your joints.

WHICH AEROBIC EXERCISE IS BEST FOR YOU?

Most people can take a brisk walk, jog, cycle, or swim. Nowadays there are devices that can be used at home or in gyms that simulate just about every type of exercise. Table 15.2 lists the best types of aerobic exercise and the approximate time required to achieve a significant training effect.

WHAT TIME OF DAY IS BEST?

The best time of day to exercise is open to debate: physiology gives the edge to the end of the day and sociology to the beginning of the day.

Exercise not only tones the body, it also relieves stress and tones the mind. Stress for most people is usually highest at the end of the day, so exercise then helps the mind as much as the muscles.

Early morning exercise, however, provides a different advantage. Any time you exercise, your brain produces natural opiates called endorphins, which elevate your mood so you become more optimistic. While they help you feel better after the day is done, they also help you start the day with an optimistic outlook. So, while evening exercise is biologically a little better for relieving stress and eliminating toxins, it does not have a great advantage.

Sociologists have learned that people who exercise in the morning are less likely to quit, because most people have more control of the early morning hours before the day's obligations take over. All you have to do is rise earlier and get started. Most studies also have shown that morning exercise makes you more efficient during the day. Whatever time of day you choose, the important thing is to exercise.

START NOW

By the time you finish reading this paragraph, you will have 100,000 new blood cells and about 14,000,000 other new cells. These cells can use the extra air you'll get through exercise to do good and be better. If you haven't been exercising, start slowly; a brisk 15-minute walk is an excellent way to start, and then work up to 40 minutes. Next, progress to brisk walking for 5 minutes, alternating with 1 minute of jogging, followed by 5 minutes of walking; continue in this manner for up to 40 minutes. A healthy person with no leg or heart problems can maintain a 12- to 15-minutes-per-mile pace for 40 minutes, or about 2½ or 3 miles. A practiced, brisk walker will do 10 minutes per mile. You can follow the same pattern with a stationary bicycle or any other device.

16

Lose Excess Weight and Don't Gain It Back

Excess weight is characteristic of affluent societies throughout the world, especially in the last decade. The United States is now the most affluent—and the most overweight—society ever. Over 50 percent of the U.S. population is overweight, and over half of these people are seriously obese (20 percent above normal weight). Over 30 percent of children in the United States are overweight.

Being overweight compromises health and longevity. It shortens life expectancy; increases heart disease and all associated risk factors; increases cancer risk; makes all illnesses worse; and slows recovery.

Stress is a major causative factor in being overweight, and at the same time the excess weight places a stress on every body system. This becomes an insidious spiral from which only the most determined can extract themselves.

Losing weight isn't easy. Over 70 percent of adults will tell you at any given time they would like to lose about ten pounds. Considering that over 50 percent are clinically overweight despite this desire, we can infer that losing weight is a difficult task. Even more difficult is keeping the weight off once it has been lost.

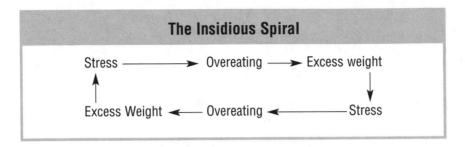

Often, people will say that their excess weight is caused by some mysterious glandular disorder. That flies in the face of scientific evidence. Some studies have shown that some overweight people do have serious problems that cause them to eat excessively; however, about 99 percent of all overweight people can lose weight and keep it off once it is lost. Blaming our glands is simply not valid.

Losing weight and keeping it off has been proven over and over to improve health and longevity. We have much to gain by getting down to and maintaining a normal weight.

THE ARITHMETIC OF EXCESS WEIGHT

A pound of body fat represents an accumulation of 3,500 excess calories; over some period of time (say a week or two), that person ate 3,500 more calories than he burned, and his efficient body stored it as fat for some future time when things wouldn't be so good. When that person loses a pound, it means that over a period of time he burned 3,500 more calories than he ate, and his body simply used those calories it had stored for lean times.

Since most adults, when asked, say they would like to lose about 10 pounds, they have to create a 35,000-calorie deficit over some reasonable period, perhaps four or six weeks. Creating a calorie deficit is just like creating a financial deficit; to do that you only need to spend more money, say, with a credit card, than you earn. To create a calorie deficit, you simply have to burn more calories than you eat. It is that simple! No matter how many "magical" diets there are, no matter how many "magic" pills, herbs, nostrums, and smooth-talking diet gurus there are, weight loss comes down to this simple fact: Create a calorie deficit and you will lose weight. Once you have lost weight, you won't gain it back—if you eat only as many calories as you burn.

CALORIES AND BASAL METABOLIC RATE

If you are overweight, it is because your body is overfat or because your lean body mass (LBM), consisting of muscles, bones, and tissues with no fat, is too low for your weight. To lose weight, you need to lose fat and gain more muscle.

Basal metabolism, the energy allocated to keeping the body functioning, burns more calories than any other bodily activity during a twenty-four-hour day. For example, a 125-pound woman can get along well on 1,800 calories each day. Of those 1,800 calories, about 1,200 go to her basal metabolism. No matter what she is doing, even sleeping, her heart beats, her temperature remains normal, her kidneys remove wastes, her brain keeps everything working, she breathes, and all the myriad body processes keep going. That's her basal metabolic rate (BMR).

You can get a good picture of your BMR by consulting Table 16.1.

Burning Excess Calories

People recognize that exercise burns calories, which is correct. However, for a 120-pound woman to burn off a 300-calorie piece of cake, she has to exercise vigorously for 83 minutes. That is 83 minutes of fast (7.5 minutes per mile) jogging or the same time on a Stairmaster or NordicTrack. It is not easy to get rid of extra calories by exercise.

Table 16.1

Approximate Basal Metabolic Rate in Calories

Height	Weight*	Calories per 24 hours					
		Age 20	Age 30	Age 40	Age 50	Age 60	Age 70
FEMALE							
5 ft 2 in	110 lb	1234	1243	1211	1176	1137	1105
	130 lb	1339	1327	1293	1255	1213	1179
	150 lb	1423	1411	1375	1335	1290	1254
5 ft 5 in	125 lb	1372	1361	1326	1287	1244	1209
	145 lb	1457	1445	1408	1366	1321	1284
	165 lb	1542	1529	1489	1446	1398	1358
5 ft 7 in	135 lb	1457	1445	1400	1366	1321	1204
	155 lb	1542	1529	1489	1446	1398	1358
	175 lb	1627	1613	1571	1525	1475	1433
MALE							
5 ft 10 in	160 lb	1819	1715	1660	1632	1573	1491
	180 lb	1915	1805	1747	1718	1656	1570
	200 lb	2011	1895	1835	1804	1739	1648
6 ft	170 lb	1896	1787	1730	1701	1639	1554
	190 lb	1992	1877	1817	1787	1722	1632
	210 lb	2088	1967	1904	1873	1805	1711
6 ft 2 in	180 lb	1992	1877	1817	1787	1722	1632
	200 lb	2088	1967	1904	1873	1805	1711
	210 lb	2145	2021	1957	1925	1855	1758

* Three weights are given for each height: the first is ideal weight, the second is overweight, the third is obese. A formula for working out your ideal weight is as follows:

Females—multiply every inch over five feet by 5 and add 100.

Males—multiply every inch over five feet by 5 and add 110.

Note: Personal BMR varies from one person to another and can depend on heredity. It may also vary according to the environment: in cold weather the metabolic rate is higher to keep you warm; in warmer weather, depending on humidity, it has a tendency to be lower. The lower your body-fat content, the higher your metabolic rate will be.

Table 16.2

Daily Energy in Two Lives

	170-pound man	130-pound woman
BMR	1787	1327
Work energy: Light (salesperson/teacher)	536	398
Energy lost to food	179	133
Exercise: Vigorous for 30 minutes	153	117
Total energy in calories	2655	1975

Some additional energy gets used simply digesting your food. For example, you probably don't gain any calories by eating celery; in fact, you likely lose some. (You also lose more calories to digestion if you are upset.) Most experts estimate this loss at about 10 percent of BMR.

The two practical examples in Table 16.2 will give you a good idea of the energy expenditure during a typical day for two people: a 170-pound man and a 130-pound woman.

DIETING DOES WORK

Just about every day a new diet comes on the market that purports to work better than every other diet. Logic tells you that if these diets worked—and most do to some extent—there must be something about losing and keeping weight off that goes beyond maintaining calorie balance.

Weight is always a complex interaction of heredity and environmental factors so subtle as to defy complete analysis. Superimposed on all that complexity are the ways every society uses food: for pleasure, conducting business, social interaction, and even family fellowship. In addition, advertising in our culture hits us from every direction, and about 95 percent of food advertising is for foods that deliver lots of calories with little nutritional value.

So, the problem with dieting is that once you've lost the weight, you must return to the world that caused you to gain weight in the first place. That is why dieters usually gain back the pounds they've lost, plus a little extra.

More frustrating yet is the rate at which weight can be lost. If a person follows a typical fad diet, say, the latest high-protein diet, he will lose a lot of weight, up to 5 percent of body weight, in the first week. After that, it comes off at about 1.5 to 2.5 pounds per week, depending on how overweight he was originally.

Therefore, losing 50 pounds, which were probably put on over a few years, takes about fifteen to twenty weeks, or four to six months. Dieting for that long requires willpower that will challenge even the most dedicated dieter.

Don't become pessimistic, however, because there is a plan that works. It is so deceptively simple that few people use it, but those who do always succeed.

Food Diaries and Fat Bags

A medical school conducted a study on two groups of people who wanted to lose weight. Members of the baseline group were asked to keep a daily food diary showing everything they ate with a notation of when and why, followed by a daily paragraph critiquing the day's eating. Members of the other group were asked to follow a carefully worked-out diet and were provided with motivators to encourage them.

After about two weeks, the diary-keeping group started losing weight at the same rate as the dieting group. Within two months the diary group's rate of loss surpassed that of the other dieters. The reason was quite simple: Without even realizing it, the diary keepers had taken control of what they were eating by recording it in the notebook and evaluating it without emotion. People know what is good for them, what is excessive, and what they should and should not eat. Once you put it in writing (and if you're not in serious denial), what you need to do becomes obvious if you have any interest in achieving good health.

The food diary must list everything you eat, as well as why you eat it, when you eat it, and any special circumstances. Pretty soon you'll start understanding why you eat what you do. The daily critique paragraph helps you see where you can do better and where to apply willpower.

Fat bags are another simple device that also helped members of the baseline group lose weight. Each person was instructed to purchase a pound of sand for each pound she wanted to lose, as well as a cloth bag, called a fat bag. For each pound that came off, a pound of sand was put in the fat bag, which was displayed prominently. Some people displayed their fat bags at work, much like people keep family photos on their desks. The fat bag is a trophy you can give yourself and show others.

It pays to join or organize a weight-loss group whose members have to "weigh in" each week. The motivation of the round of applause you get for each lost pound, added to the fat bag trophy, is enough to boost anyone's willpower.

The bottom line is simple: gain control of your emotions and eat sensibly so you will lose the weight you must and keep it off permanently.

17

Manage K-Factor and Control Salt in Your Diet

Managing K-factor and dietary salt is a simple, effective way to directly and indirectly reduce the amount of stress placed on your body, by

- improving cardiovascular health,
- placing less stress on your kidneys,
- lowering blood pressure,
- reducing fluid retention, and
- making weight control easier.

As your health improves, so does your ability to handle stress.

WHAT IS K-FACTOR?

K-factor is the ratio of sodium to potassium in our diets. When the average dietary K-factor is 3 or more, the incidence of hypertension is very low, less than 2 percent of the population and mostly restricted to very overweight people. As the ratio approaches 1, the incidence of high blood pressure in the population increases dramatically, as shown in Table 17.1.

Table 17.1	
K-Factor and High Blood Pressure in a Population	
K-Factor	**Incidence of High Blood Pressure**
4.0 or more	2%
1.1	26%
0.4	33%

Sodium and potassium are the two major electrolytes in the body. A third, chloride, is also essential. Potassium is very plentiful in natural, unprocessed foods; in contrast, sodium and chloride are very scarce in natural foods. Our kidneys not only eliminate waste materials, they're also marvelously designed to conserve sodium and chloride because those elements were once so scarce. For example, in the early Roman Empire soldiers were paid a salt ration, much the same way early gold miners were paid with gold dust. The word *salary* actually comes from the Latin for "salt ration." In a few isolated places in the world, salt still has this value. When there is excess sodium and chloride salt in the diet, the kidneys conserve it. After all, they've been doing this for over three million years. Through a complex series of interactions, this conservation of sodium and chloride causes an increase in blood volume. Increased blood volume causes high blood pressure.

A correct K-factor can't be restored by simply adding potassium back to the diet to offset the sodium, because the total amount of salt, more specifically sodium, must be considered. People with high blood pressure absolutely must control their sodium intake, salt consumption, and K-factor. Anyone who lives, works, or commutes in a stressful occupation or environment should also control their dietary K-factor.

CONTROLLING SALT AND SODIUM

Do not eat a food that provides over 75 milligrams of sodium chloride, and eat no meal that provides over 200 milligrams. If you follow this rule your diet will contain less than 800 milligrams of sodium chloride and much less than 2,000 milligrams of salt daily. Some foods, such as milk, contain natural sodium. These foods are generally all right. Natural sodium still adds up, but it is not salt (sodium chloride), and the body tolerates it better.

Table 17.2 summarizes the sodium content, potassium content, and K-factor of selected foods.

Table 17.2			
The Nutritional Cost of Food Processing			
Food	Sodium (mg. per serving)	Potassium (mg. per serving)	K-Factor
Beef	44	311	7.00
Hot dog (all beef)	461	71	0.15
Chicken breast	80	360	4.50
Fast-food or frozen and breaded chicken	1012	360	0.40
Corn (fresh)	11	219	20.00
Corn flakes	351	26	0.07
Canned corn	680	219	0.30
Shredded Wheat (Nabisco)	6	150	25.00

Note the effect that processing has on a food's K-factor. Beef is a good example. Most cuts provide about 44 milligrams of sodium and 311 milligrams of potassium; divide 311 by 44, and you get a K-factor of about 7. That is excellent! Now do the same for the "all beef" hot dog. Go down the list to corn. As you can see, fresh corn is great, but any processing lessens its value immediately.

Reading ingredients lists is the only way to avoid sodium in processed food. If salt appears in the list, the food should be avoided, even if the product name or other labeling implies that it is somehow low in salt.

Some processed foods, however, are naturally low in sodium, such as Shredded Wheat and pasta. At the bottom of the nutritional label of processed and packaged foods is a listing of the sodium and potassium content of each serving. Divide potassium by sodium to get the K-factor. Never eat a food that has a K-factor of less than 3! If the nutrition label doesn't have the sodium and potassium content, and you have the slightest doubt, avoid the product.

There are a number of salt-free ways you can spice up foods you prepare yourself. Excellent salt substitutes include Tabasco sauce, horseradish, Tone Brothers Perc seasonings, and Mrs. Dash seasonings.

Sodium and Water

Tap water and bottled water sometimes contain too much sodium. Often the sodium is salt (sodium chloride). To determine the salt content of your tap water, ask your municipal government. The salt content of bottled water should be indicated on the label. Do some calculations. You should drink about 64 ounces of water daily; that is a little over 2 quarts. If the water doesn't supply more than 25 milligrams of sodium per quart, it is all right. Even if you don't drink any water, you get it from beverages and foods. Remember, you should be drinking a minimum of 32 ounces of water daily.

GETTING SUFFICIENT POTASSIUM

Eat natural foods, and your potassium intake will take care of itself. You require about 3,000 milligrams of potassium daily. If you eat natural foods with a good variety of vegetables, fruits, grains, and cereals, you needn't worry. Foods that are especially rich in potassium are bananas, avocados, artichokes, and fresh or frozen beans (not canned). You shouldn't use potassium supplements unless you are instructed to do so by a physician to compensate for the regular use of a prescription diuretic.

A good source of information on sodium and potassium is *Bowes and Church's Food Values of Portions Commonly Used,* by Jean A. T. Pennington, Ph.D., R.D. My book *The High Blood Pressure Relief Diet* also contains data and information on foods and menu planning, as well as an extensive reading list.

18

Take a Basic Multiple Vitamin and Mineral Supplement Daily

To function normally—and to handle stress well—your body requires nineteen vitamins and minerals daily in addition to protein, fat, carbohydrates, and fiber. These requirements are expressed in terms of the recommended daily intake (RDI). Vitamins and most minerals are required in very small (trace) quantities. For example, every day you need just 400 micrograms (400 millionths of a gram) of the B vitamin folic acid. In contrast, calcium is required in comparatively large amounts, ranging from 1,000 milligrams (1 gram) for most women up to about age fifty; after that age the need increases to 1,200 milligrams. Magnesium's requirement is somewhat midway; you need 200 to 400 milligrams ($\frac{4}{10}$ gram) daily. With the exception of calcium (discussed in detail in chapter 19) and magnesium, all your vitamin and mineral needs can be packed into a single large tablet. I don't believe in leaving anything to chance, so I recommend you supplement your diet to avoid any possible marginal deficiencies.

Use a supplement that provides the vitamins and minerals in the amounts listed in Table 18.1. Most supplements contain values within 10 to 20 percent of those listed here. It is important that your supplement contains all these vitamins and minerals and that you take it daily.

Few products satisfy all these criteria. Usually the product you select will have less calcium and magnesium. If so, don't worry, because you should take extra calcium anyway. Most likely, your diet already contains excess phosphorus and about 20 percent of the magnesium you need. If the product you select comes within 20 percent of the calcium, magnesium, and phosphorus levels listed in Table 18.1, it is fine. Don't select a supplement that varies in these three areas by more than that amount.

IS MORE BETTER?

Most vitamins are safe at ten or more times the RDI, so if you choose to do as I do and take some extra, you don't have to worry—you're not harming yourself. Recent studies of elderly people indicate that our needs increase as we get older, so taking more than the RDI is undoubtedly beneficial.

COMMON QUESTIONS ABOUT SUPPLEMENT USE

Question: Aren't excess vitamins and minerals just excreted, creating expensive urine?

Answer: Especially when you're under stress, but even if you're starving, your body will lose some vitamins and minerals daily through excretion. Under those conditions, your urine is truly "expensive." If your blood levels of nutrients are high, your urine levels will also be higher; that is normal human physiology.

Table 18.1

Basic Supplements

Nutrient Vitamin	Amount per Tablet*	Percent U.S. RDI
Vitamin A (as beta carotene)	2,500 I.U.** (500 mcg. RE***)	50
Vitamin D	200 I.U. (5 mcg.)	50
Vitamin E	15 I.U. (5 mg. alpha-tocopherol equivalents)	50
Vitamin C	30 mg.	50
Folic acid	0.2 mg.	50
Thiamin (B₁)	0.75 mg.	50
Riboflavin (B₂)	0.86 mg.	50
Niacin	10 mg.	50
Vitamin B₆	1 mg.	50
Vitamin B₁₂	3 mcg.	50
Biotin	0.15 mg. (150 mcg.)	50
Pantothenic acid	5 mg.	50

Nutrient Mineral

Calcium	125 mg.	25
Phosphorus	180 mg.	40
Iodine	75 mcg.	50
Iron	9 mg.	50
Magnesium	50 mg.	12.5
Copper	1 mg.	50
Zinc	1 mg.	50
Selenium	50 mcg.	****
Manganese	0.5 mg.	****
Chromium	50 mcg.	****
Molybdenum	30 mcg.	****

    * Two tablets provide 100 percent U.S. RDI for all nutrients except calcium, phosphorus, and magnesium.
   ** International Units.
  *** Microgram retinol equivalents.
 **** U.S. RDI not established.

Question: Isn't it expensive to take vitamins and minerals?

Answer: In our society, about one dollar per person is spent daily on soft drinks. Is that wasteful? Expensive is meaningful only by comparison. The multiple vitamin and mineral supplement costs less than 25 cents daily. Is your health worth twenty-five cents a day?

Question: A salesperson I know sells a brand of vitamins not available in stores. He says they're better and are all natural, but they're quite expensive. Should I use them?

Answer: Just about all vitamins are made by five companies worldwide. Every atom in each vitamin is as natural as the atom in any other vitamin. My advice is to go with a good brand name because name-brand firms have the most to lose if something goes wrong and therefore usually have the best quality control.

Question: I notice some companies have products that are targeted to specific age groups. I can understand supplements for children, but what about those aimed at seniors?

Answer: If the supplement supplies at least what is listed in Table 18.1, it is fine. A little more won't hurt and can actually help.

19

Get Enough Calcium and Magnesium

While very little research has been conducted on the role of stress in calcium loss, there seems to be a connection. People under emotional stress lose more calcium. Inactivity is another stressor that definitely causes calcium loss. It is nature's way of saying, "If you don't use it, you lose it!" Exercise is absolutely essential for effective calcium utilization.

Table 19.1

Food Sources for 1,000 Milligrams of Calcium

Food	Amount	Calories	Comments
Cheddar cheese	5 oz.	560	Fat is bad
Low-fat cottage cheese	5.2 oz.	1,066	Too much fat and sodium
Skim milk	27 fl. oz. (3⅓ 8-oz. glasses)	290	Good source
Low-fat yogurt	19 oz.	466	Good source

Government nutrition and food analyses indicate that calcium is generally lacking in most people's diets. In fact, many experts both use and recommend calcium supplements. In addition to the difficulty of obtaining adequate dietary calcium, many lifestyle habits, such as use of caffeine, excess sodium intake, and lack of exercise, cause calcium loss. Therefore, common sense dictates that one take 400 to 600 milligrams of calcium daily as insurance. Table 19.1 shows some food sources for calcium.

Unlike many nutrients, calcium shortfalls are additive. That means that if you fall short for a year or two, say, when you're a teenager, and then you do it again during your childbearing years, your bones will be less dense than if you hadn't fallen short at all. Below-normal bone density is the condition called *osteoporosis,* which causes much suffering and even death for the elderly.

Bone calcium loss is accelerated by caffeine (coffee, tea, soft drinks), excess meat, salt, and inadequate exercise. However, much clinical research in many countries has proven that bone density can be restored by using calcium supplements. If you drink more than two cups of coffee or its equivalent in tea or soft drinks, take an extra 200 milligrams daily.

CALCIUM AND WOMEN'S HEALTH

Adult women require 1,000 milligrams of calcium each day up to about age fifty; after that, most nutritionists believe that calcium intake should be increased to 1,200 or 1,500 milligrams. Milk, yogurt, and cheese are the most common sources of calcium; however, a one-cup serving of broccoli or spinach provides the calcium of half a glass of milk, together with other nutrients. Ask yourself if you consume sufficient dairy products and calcium-rich foods each day. Common sense suggests you should use calcium supplements (up to about 1,000 milligrams of calcium daily).

WHAT ABOUT MEN?

Because men don't bear children and have different hormones, they have only about 60 to 80 percent of the calcium requirement that women have. Once past about age twenty-one, however, they begin to fall short in their calcium intake. Then, as they age, they need almost as much as women. Consequently, although risk of calcium deficiency in women is emphasized more, men could do well by following the advice given to women.

MAGNESIUM: A PARTNER WITH CALCIUM

Most dietary analyses indicate that we usually do not get enough of the mineral magnesium, as well as calcium. Since 200 to 400 milligrams of magnesium are required daily, a good policy is to take a calcium supplement that also contains some magnesium.

Some self-proclaimed experts advise a specific calcium-magnesium ratio for good health. However, a brilliant scientist, Dr. Mildred Seelig, conducted a careful study of adult needs for calcium and magnesium and proved that once you achieve an intake of about 400 milligrams of magnesium daily, the body can use calcium very effectively, and there is no need to get more magnesium.

COMMON QUESTIONS ABOUT CALCIUM

Question: Will calcium cause kidney stones?

Answer: No! Extensive research in both men and women has proven that calcium actually reduces the risk of kidney stone formation. The same research indicated that people who have a tendency toward stone formation should drink more fluids.

Question: Should I take 1,000 to 1,500 milligrams of calcium at one time?

Answer: No, calcium will be absorbed more efficiently if you space it out, taking it two or three times daily. For example, if you take 1,200 milligrams daily, take 600 milligrams in the morning and 600 in the evening, or take 400 milligrams three times a day.

Question: When should I take calcium?

Answer: Calcium is absorbed best when it is taken with food. The carbohydrates in food seem to facilitate calcium absorption. So, take calcium supplements at mealtime.

20

Increase Your Vitamin Intake: B-Complex, C, and E

Taking a multiple vitamin and mineral supplement, as advised in chapter 18, should provide an adequate amount of all the necessary vitamins and minerals if you're average and eat a fairly good diet. When you live or work in a stressful environment, however, a case can be made for more of the B vitamins and vitamins C and E. If you engage in active, aggressive physical activity, which is physical stress, albeit controlled, more of these nutrients are required. Review your environment and decide for yourself:

- Do you live under stressful conditions?
- Do you work in a stressful environment?
- Do you commute over thirty minutes in heavy traffic?
- Are you exposed to a smoky or polluted environment?
- Are you exposed to solvent fumes?
- Do you take patented or prescription medication regularly?
- Do you engage in intense physical activity for over thirty minutes daily?

Answering yes to any of these questions could mean you need more B-complex and the antioxidant vitamins, so read on.

B-COMPLEX VITAMINS

All metabolism requires the seven common B vitamins. Several avenues of research have shown that under physical stress, especially physical injury, the body needs more of these nutrients. When people are under emotional stress, they often feel more relaxed when they take B-complex vitamins in amounts over and above the multiple vitamin and mineral supplement already described and recommended.

Many experts call the B-complex vitamins "stress relievers," and some physicians prescribe them when people are under stress, especially when they feel depressed. Depression is often a stress symptom that causes insomnia and sets a cycle of increasing stress in motion. The simplest way to rule out B-complex deficiency as a factor in stress is to take an extra amount as a daily supplement.

Table 20.1	
The B-Complex Vitamins	
Vitamin	**RDI**
Thiamin, B_1	1.5 mg
Riboflavin, B_2	1.7 mg
Niacin	19 mg
Pyridoxal phosphate, B_6	2.0 mg
B_{12}	2.0 mcg
Biotin	60 mcg
Folic acid	200 mcg

If you take a B-complex supplement, make sure your supplement is balanced with respect to the RDI given in Table 20.1.

Questions About B-Complex Vitamins

Question: I found a B-complex supplement that claims it is balanced for stress. It contains much more B_6 and very little biotin. Is it better?

Answer: No! There is no "stress balance." Those products usually provide large quantities of the inexpensive (B_6) vitamins and very little of the expensive (biotin) and have absolutely no scientific foundation.

Question: I found a product that provides zinc and magnesium in addition to the B vitamins. It is called a "stress formula." Is this a good product for stress?

Answer: The use of zinc to alleviate stress was based on a study of people who were burned over at least 40 percent of their bodies. These people were clearly under stress, but their zinc loss was a result of fluid loss. It had nothing to do with emotional stress.

VITAMIN C

Research suggests that the RDI of vitamin C should be about 100 to 150 milligrams under most conditions. If you live or work in a smoky environment or must commute long hours in a car while in traffic, you need more vitamin C than provided by the RDI.

When your body is placed under stress, its vitamin C level drops because your body is using more vitamin C to counter the attack; however, you don't make vitamin C. An important change is the drop of the vitamin C level in leukocytes, the white blood cells, when you're under physical or emotional stress. This drop in vitamin C explains why a chill (physical stress) often brings on a cold. You get a chill, which stresses your whole body, so the vitamin C level drops throughout your body. Leukocytes are the first line of defense. When the leukocytes and other immune materials called antibodies drop below normal because of inadequate vitamin C, cold viruses can multiply. Vitamin C speeds the production of immune materials, which is why vitamin C makes the cold less severe. In vitamin C deficiency, the number of these cells drops as much as 25 percent, and those that survive lose as much as 25 percent of their ability to attack foreign agents. It adds up to a 50 percent loss.

We can make a case for between 100 and 500 milligrams of vitamin C daily. These levels can be achieved by starting your day with orange juice and then making sure you get at least four or more servings of fruits and vegetables.

People who regularly use aspirin or other nonsteroidal anti-inflammatory drugs (NSAIDs) require more vitamin C, as do people who use steroids. In both cases, an extra 500 milligrams of vitamin C daily will cover the requirement.

Physical stress as determined by testing athletes increases the vitamin C requirement. To translate an athlete's need to the average person in a stressful job or to the homemaker with several children is not scientifically valid. However, taking up to 1,000 milligrams of vitamin C daily does have some benefits and no negative side effects. Therefore, how much to take is a personal decision.

If you decide on a special vitamin C supplement, select one that provides 500 milligrams per tablet. Should you decide you need 1,000 milligrams daily, take one 500-milligram tablet twice daily, in the morning and evening.

VITAMIN E

Age spots (*fleurs de cimitière* in French) appear on the backs of our hands, on our faces, and on other parts of the body. Though you can't see them, they also appear on the internal organs.

Age spots are accumulations of pigment involving rancid oils, called lipofuscin. French folk wisdom holds that wheat germ or wheat germ oil prevents age spots. The only nutritional way to prevent the onset of age spots is with vitamin E, and wheat germ oil happens to be the best natural source of vitamin E. This folk wisdom goes right to the heart of vitamins E's function: preventing the oxidation of essential oils in the body. In this way, vitamin E actually slows the aging process.

If you want to get 50 milligrams of vitamin E daily, you will need to take a supplement that contains at least 30 milligrams, and you'd be better off taking one that provides 40 milligrams. One advantage of taking extra vitamin E is that it is retained by your body. Therefore, if you took a 400-I.U. supplement or 240 milligrams once weekly, that would maintain a running average of about 50 milligrams daily if you eat a good diet. Since almost all of the most concentrated sources of vitamin E are very high in calories, a vitamin E supplement will more easily fit into your calorie limits.

21

Use Fiber as a Stress Fighter

Bowel regularity is essential to good health, and as we've seen, good health is an essential part of stress reduction. Dietary fiber, the food component for regularity, ranks with vitamins and minerals as an essential, albeit often forgotten, nutrient—forgotten because from a relatively early age, most people don't get sufficient fiber. This means increased risk of fiber-related diseases, which include diverticulosis, cardiovascular diseases, cancer, high blood pressure, and many others. Only 5 percent of adults meet their daily dietary fiber requirement. Most people get only 50 percent of their daily dietary fiber.

Our bodies produce many materials that are eliminated in urine by way of the gallbladder or through the intestine itself; the system should have available adequate dietary fiber to bind up these materials and flush them from the body. Generally, this means getting 25 to 35 grams of dietary fiber each day from carbohydrate-rich foods and fiber supplements.

WHAT DOES FIBER DO?

Fiber is like a brush that, in addition to moving things along, can selectively bind unwanted materials and remove them from the system. There are about five or six types of fiber, all of which have properties we require, and a varied diet provides them all. Of course, selective supplementation helps.

Hard fiber, the type found in wheat bran, is the "water carrier" that helps to produce regularity. It gives good stool consistency. This fiber is found in all plant foods, but mostly in high-fiber cereals, grains, most vegetables, beans, and tubers such as potatoes. You can't eat too much of these foods, and the results will be obvious as you increase them in your diet.

In contrast to hard fiber, the soluble forms of fiber, such as pectin, gums, saponins, and others, are the best at selective adsorption. For example, pectin helps to reduce cholesterol and blood fat by binding the bile acids produced by our livers from cholesterol and removing them in our stools. Oat bran does it even better, and guar gum better yet. Soluble fiber also binds the cholesterol and fat that we get in our diet and helps to carry them through the system.

There is evidence that the soluble dietary fiber from fruits and vegetables can help to remove unhelpful by-products of metabolism, which helps relieve stress. It appears that some materials produced by the body and secreted into the intestine by the gallbladder, in the absence of sufficient fiber, are reabsorbed and thereby act as antagonists and cause problems. The results of intestinal bypass surgery reveal that the microflora of the intestine also removes toxic by-products.

FIBER FROM FOOD

An easy way to get enough fiber is to begin each day with high-fiber cereal. Many excellent cereals are available: Fiber One, All-Bran, Bran Buds, bran flakes, corn bran, oat bran, oatmeal, and barley, to name a few. Add unprocessed bran to pancakes or waffles. Eat fruit on cereal, in pancakes, or plain; eat fruit, vegetables, grains, and tubers at each meal. As your fiber intake improves, your bowels will become more regular.

SHOULD YOU USE FIBER SUPPLEMENTS?

I'm often asked, "How do I know I'm getting enough fiber?" My answer is: "You should have an easy bowel movement every twenty-four hours. The stools should be well formed and their color should be light brown; preferably about 10 percent will float."

If your stools don't fit that profile, start using a good fiber supplement. Fiber supplements are usually made from psyllium husks and are often sold as "natural vegetable laxatives" under store-brand names. Mix about one or two heaping teaspoonfuls or a full tablespoon with water, and drink it about thirty minutes before a meal.

An ideal fiber supplement has the following ingredients: psyllium husks, apple fiber, acacia gum, guar gum, oat bran, and a few ingredients to improve taste and dissolvability. However, it is acceptable to use a fiber supplement that contains only psyllium husks. Any supplement should provide from 3 to 4 grams of fiber per tablespoon.

A DAY WITH 35 GRAMS OF FIBER

Most people have difficulty understanding how 25 to 35 grams of fiber intake daily is achieved, so I've prepared Table 21.1. This "Day of Fiber" exceeds what most people require; for example, a 125-pound woman does fine on 25 to 30 grams daily, while her 200-pound husband needs 35 grams.

Also recognize that this guide allows for many substitutions. For instance, beans and rice are an excellent protein entrée that also

Table 21.1

A Day with 35 Grams of Fiber

Food Item	Soluble	Insoluble	Total	Calories
Breakfast				
Bran flakes	1.0	4.0	5.0	121
(with ½ cup skim milk)				93
½ grapefruit	0.6	1.1	1.7	39
Snack				
Banana	0.6	1.4	2.0	105
Lunch				
2 slices wheat bread	0.6	2.2	2.8	122
Corn (½ cup)	1.7	2.2	3.9	89
Broccoli	1.6	2.3	3.9	23
Peach (dessert)	0.6	1.0	1.6	37
Snack				
Apple	0.8	2.0	2.8	81
Dinner				
Brussels sprouts	1.6	2.3	3.9	30
Small salad	1.6	2.2	3.8	50
Potato	0.7	1.0	1.7	200
Melon (dessert)	0.4	0.6	1.0	130
Snack				
Pear (crispy)	0.5	2.0	2.5	98
Total	**12.3**	**24.3**	**35.6**	**1218**

Other foods eaten during the day:	Calories
Yogurt, low-fat	228
Fish	150
Turkey slices	100
Spreads and condiments	100
Total calories	**578**
Total daily calories	**1796**

* This day is designed to provide enough fiber with flexibility. There's room to have other desserts or accompaniments, such as wine, up to 1,800 calories for women and 2,200 calories for men.

provides fiber. That combination could easily substitute for a luncheon sandwich.

You cannot get too much dietary fiber. In the past thirty years, I've never observed a study in which people have gotten too much dietary fiber, and that includes those in which the volunteers ingested as much as 90 grams daily.

Fiber Tips

- Fiber can help relieve stress and contribute to general health.
- Fiber is obtained from cereals, grains, fruits, and vegetables. It is also available in supplement form.
- There are many types of fiber and all are important; therefore, eat a variety.
- Water is necessary as both a nutrient and a teamworker with fiber. Drink lots of water.

22

Avoid Excess Alcohol

Alcohol probably ranks above eating as the most common stress reliever. While modest alcohol consumption—for example, a glass of red wine with dinner—is a healthy habit, excessive alcohol consumption, or alcohol abuse, is a deadly practice. Alcohol abuse can cause serious physical as well as social problems, because it destroys your body from within.

Alcohol is a toxin; it crosses the blood-brain barrier and at high enough levels can cause the brain to stop functioning. When a person eats while drinking, his blood alcohol doesn't rise as rapidly. (That is one good reason to always drink socially and take food at the same time.) However, you can't rely on food to prevent the effects of alcohol.

Because alcohol is a toxin, the body detoxifies alcohol as quickly as possible by metabolizing (burning) it to become carbon dioxide and water. In fact, when alcohol enters the blood, the liver stops metabolizing everything else and focuses all its attention and effort on eliminating the alcohol. That means that any fat or carbohydrate circulating in the blood will have to wait for processing until the alcohol is reduced to a manageable level. Excess blood fat is first stored in the liver; sugar simply stays in the blood, and its level continues to rise. This is why excessive alcohol consumption on a regular basis causes fatty deposits in the liver, which leads to cirrhosis of the liver.

The excess sugar is converted to fat and often winds up in the same place. In addition, the excess sugar can cause a similar excess of insulin production, and when the alcohol is gone, the blood sugar drops. The drinker usually goes for more alcohol when that happens.

Low blood sugar is one of the worst messages the brain can receive. It is a signal that the energy necessary to keep its critical processes going is dwindling. Anxiety follows that signal, which manifests itself in no time as irritability and erratic behavior. When blood sugar drops, the person usually eats more food or drinks more alcohol—neither of which is a good idea. This proves the old saying about alcohol: Moderation is the only way to go!

People who drink socially consume, on average, about 2 percent of their calories in alcoholic beverages, with no adverse effects. Active people who are physically fit can usually handle much more than 2 percent of calories; probably 4 to 5 percent. If you're 5 feet 5 inches tall, you probably burn about 1,800 calories daily; if you're 6 feet tall, you use 2,200 calories or more daily. Two percent of these levels is 35 to 45 calories daily. One and a half ounces of whiskey contain 105 calories, and a 3½-ounce glass of wine has 75 calories of alcohol. What that translates to is a few glasses of wine or beer every week, probably on weekends or occasionally with dinner.

Since the liver can process about 1 to 2 ounces of alcohol per hour, the social drinking described above is no problem. Indeed, in recent years scientists have found that one glass of wine daily or even a mixed drink or beer reduces the risk of heart disease by helping to elevate a fraction of the "good" cholesterol. Social drinking is not a bad habit and actually has some health benefits.

HOW MUCH IS SAFE?

A woman about 5 feet 6 inches tall who weighs 120 to 130 pounds should be able to consume daily a glass or two of wine, a mixed drink containing 1½ ounces of whiskey, or a couple of beers. At a cocktail party, she should not exceed one alcoholic drink or glass of wine per hour. Larger people can drink proportionately more; for example, a 6-foot 3-inch, 190-pound man can probably safely consume a third as much. He could drink about one and a half drinks per hour.

Any dinner, office, or cocktail party can easily provide a week's worth of calories from alcohol. Two glasses of wine at a holiday celebration is hardly excessive, but keep in mind that most adults exceed their legal limit to drive if they consume three drinks within one and a half hours.

Alcohol consumed excessively (more than a drink per hour), particularly at lunch, can cause trouble during the remainder of the day. That is because it forces the body to set other caloric materials, namely sugar and fat, aside while it metabolizes the alcohol to carbon dioxide and water.

This type of drinking causes blood sugar shifts and encourages fatty deposits in the liver. A drop in blood sugar increases irritability, which usually drives the person to seek stimulants, more alcohol, or even candy. Often, doctors, not fully understanding what is going on, will encourage people who feel down or irritable in the afternoon to suck on hard candy. Sucking on the candy keeps the blood sugar up but is simply hiding the problem, while speeding the emergence of Type 2 diabetes, liver difficulties, and even periodontal trouble.

People sometimes think that taking extra B vitamins as supplements will speed the body's process of eliminating alcohol because the B vitamins are critical to alcohol metabolism. This reasoning, however, is faulty. Drinking alcohol too rapidly makes the alcohol and its by-products build up in your body faster than they can be passed out; you'll feel lousy until they're gone regardless of the amount of vitamin B in your system.

Exercise helps hasten alcohol's elimination from the body because it speeds up metabolism. However, alcohol makes it harder to exercise. Who goes to a gym after a three-martini lunch?

A hangover is usually the result of dehydration caused by excessive alcohol consumption and the elevated blood sugar that often follows. Together, these often cause fitful sleep and a severe headache the following morning.

Some people claim that drinking water when they have a hangover makes them tipsy; it's really water intoxication that their dehydrated brain is experiencing as it returns to its normal hydration level. Drinking one glass of water for every drink prevents most of these problems, but decreasing the booze is the best approach overall.

23

Eat for Stable Blood Sugar

When blood sugar drops and a person becomes hypoglycemic (has low blood sugar), stress follows quickly, even in a nonstressful environment. Whenever blood sugar drops below a natural boundary built into our physiology, it is nature's signal to the brain that its major, often only, energy source is drying up. The brain panics. You can compare this to an unexpected, severe gasoline shortage in a city just before a major holiday.

Outward anxiety follows low blood sugar because the brain is distressed; this anxiety manifests as irritability, tenseness, fear, erratic behavior, and even incoherence. If blood sugar drops low enough, a person can pass out. In these cases, the person is often erroneously advised to eat more snacks, and may be told to keep candy around. Don't follow this advice; instead, follow the tips for healthy daily eating on page 126 in this chapter.

Dietary carbohydrates—that means everything from carrots, apples, and pasta to any highly sugared foods or snacks, including soft drinks and even the sugar in your coffee—all become blood glucose, or blood sugar. For a demonstration of the amount and sources of sugar in a modern diet, do the following: Fill a 6-ounce juice glass heaping full of table sugar so the sugar starts spilling over; that's the amount of sugar the average person takes in each day. Now take out 1 tablespoon; that is the amount most people consciously add to their food, usually in coffee or tea and on cereal. The rest is found in the foods we purchase and eat daily. You'll find it on the ingredients lists of processed foods as sugar, corn syrup, corn sweeteners, corn syrup solids, glucose, fructose, and fruit sugar. Learn to read ingredients lists and you will soon realize just how much sugar you eat.

Blood sugar is important. Over our three million or more years of development, the brain has learned to rely on blood sugar for energy. In a twenty-four-hour day, about 20 percent of the circulating blood glucose will be used by the brain for energy. In a good diet the body holds blood sugar within a very liberal, yet consistent range. However, people can really mess up nature's blood sugar control system by the food they eat and cause blood sugar to swing up and down like a child's yo-yo.

WHY BLOOD SUGAR DROPS

Insulin, a hormone released by a specialized part of the pancreas, allows each of our thirteen trillion living cells to use glucose. It is as if each of these cells has a door that lets glucose in, and insulin is nature's key that unlocks that door. Lots of insulin causes all doors to open and even stay open, and when they do, blood sugar drops rapidly because insulin enters so many cells.

When you eat foods with lots of sugar and little or no fiber, the sugar is released very quickly after it leaves the stomach for the small intestine and gets absorbed into the blood while it's still in the topmost part of the intestine. For example, a soft drink has about 2 tablespoons of sugar and no fiber, so the sugar is rapidly absorbed as soon as it leaves the stomach. This rapid movement of sugar into the blood is a signal that lots of sugar is on its way, and much insulin is released so the expected sugar load can be metabolized.

Seldom is the exact amount of insulin produced to meet the need. More often than not, excess insulin is produced. If other natural foods are being eaten at the same time, a serious blood sugar drop is not experienced because fiber slows carbohydrate release, and the insulin is used more effectively. However, many people produce excess insulin whenever the sugar load exceeds their threshold, and hypoglycemia results.

When blood sugar drops, the panic and anxiety produced is actually a primitive signal telling the person to eat, or take stimulants such as coffee, alcohol, or cigarettes. People with low blood sugar often behave strangely or unpleasantly until they take in something that relieves the problem.

The smart person simply follows a diet that will keep her blood sugar within the normal range. This eliminates one stress source, and even better, it helps prevent overreaction to the stress that always follows anxiety. Stable blood sugar similarly allows a person to cope calmly with stress.

Eating to maintain normal blood sugar is simple: follow a diet high in complex carbohydrates with the correct amount of protein and not too much fat. Sound difficult? It isn't if you simply eat for bulk, avoid sugar, seek out high-fiber foods, and use fiber supplements sensibly.

Compare an apple to a piece of chocolate. Both deliver about 150 calories. You can swallow the chocolate without even chewing, but no one can swallow an apple whole. That's what bulk means. Select vegetable foods and fruits that are fresh and require chewing. Learn to make them your snacks.

GUIDELINES FOR A LOW–BLOOD SUGAR DIET

- *Vegetables:* minimum three servings daily, preferably five. A serving is ½ cup of chopped vegetables or a floret of broccoli, a medium carrot, and so on.

- *Fruit:* minimum two servings daily, preferably four. A serving is a medium apple, an orange, or a half cup of berries.
- *Cereal:* eat one that delivers a minimum of 5 grams of fiber per serving daily.
- *Grains:* minimum six servings daily, preferably more. A serving is ½ cup of corn, whole grain rice, wheat, pasta, or two slices of whole grain bread.
- *Snacks:* the best snack food available in all supermarkets is small carrots that are prewashed and packaged.
- *Beverages:* avoid all sugared beverages. Learn to use whole-pulp fruit juice. Read the ingredients list, and remember that corn sweeteners, high fructose corn syrup, and corn sugars are all names for sugar. If you have an alcoholic beverage, always accompany it with food, avoid having alcohol with highly sugared foods such as desserts, and always drink in moderation. (Read chapter 22, "Avoid Excess Alcohol.")

Protein-Rich Foods

Have you ever noticed that if you eat a couple of eggs for breakfast, you'll feel satisfied all morning, especially if you have toast and juice with the eggs? There is a reason for this, which can be used to your advantage.

Eggs are an excellent source of protein, and with the toast and juice, the protein from the eggs is combined with the carbohydrates and even some sugar. The body uses carbohydrates for energy first; then, when that is used up, say, well into the morning, some of the amino acids are used for energy, albeit more slowly, and even the fat that is found in the egg yolk.

So, the protein actually provides a secondary source of energy which doesn't call for any insulin production. This energy can be correctly called "stamina" because it comes on later and keeps a person going.

Now, don't run out and eat two eggs every morning. If you eat a good high-fiber cereal breakfast with milk, or better, a soy beverage, you'll be getting some protein that helps keep you going. This also explains why, when your blood sugar drops, an apple and a piece of cheese is a good pick-me-up. The apple acts quickly and the cheese keeps you going.

Avoid High-Fat Meals and Snacks

Athletes learn early that high-fat foods make them sluggish. Fat requires more oxygen for metabolism and takes energy-yielding oxygen, which is then used inefficiently, to metabolize the fat. So, athletes learn to rely on carbohydrates for energy. The body uses a 50:50 ratio of carbohydrate to fat in a long event, such as a marathon. Everyone can take a lesson from the athletic experience because it has its counterpart in the mental energy we all require. If you want your mind to be alert, learn to enjoy high–complex carbohydrate foods and avoid fat. This enables your brain to function at an optimum level.

Avoid protein sources that are high in fat. Seek out entrées such as fish and lean red meat, and avoid processed meats. Processed meats, including turkey bologna, are usually high in fat.

Fiber Supplements

A simple way to modulate how sugar crosses the intestinal barrier is to make sure it is enrobed in fiber. Fiber is why an apple or orange, which has the same amount of sugar as a candy bar, does not cause a "sugar rush" followed by a "sugar letdown"; the sugar crosses the intestinal barrier much more slowly. The fiber slows the sugar release and helps move it farther along the intestinal tract. This causes a slower absorption and consequently a more moderate insulin release by the pancreas.

Daily Eating to Maintain Normal Blood Sugar

Always Eat Breakfast!
High-fiber cereal with fruit
Orange juice

Midmorning Snack (Break)
(In descending order of preference, from best to worst)
Prepackaged carrots
Apple or other fruit
Bran muffins

Lunch
Two vegetables and/or salad
Fish, chicken, or other low-fat meat
Vegetarian dish, such as pizza and/or beans

Afternoon Snack
(In descending order of preference, from best to worst)
Prepackaged carrots
Fruit, such as apple, pear, or orange
Bran muffin

Stimulant Beverages (with caffeine)
(In descending order of preference, from best to worst)
Tea, plain black with milk
Coffee, made moderately strong (about 100 milligrams of caffeine per cup)
Diet caffeinated beverages
Regular caffeinated beverages

IF YOU'RE HYPOGLYCEMIC . . .

Some people have an unfortunate, probably hereditary, tendency to overproduce insulin. It seems that if they just "look at sugar," their pancreas squirts out insulin and they become hypoglycemic. Worse yet, when these people are older, they often develop a type of diabetes called adult onset or Type 2 diabetes. Characteristically, they are often overweight, even obese, because they snack so often. These people have a tendency to be overweight because they eat the normal three meals and snack regularly as well. They also tend to eat highly sugared foods because these provide the quickest relief from the anxiety that low blood sugar produces.

A simple take-control strategy is to stop eating large meals and switch to a type of eating called "grazing." "Grazers" eat lots of small meals; in fact, they eat all day long and use sensible fiber supplements. They follow the same diet as people with normal insulin production; however, they simply have smaller portions and try to eat more often.

Although a hypoglycemic should be very cautious with cheese because it has lots of fat calories, it makes an excellent snack. As a rule, if you eat an ounce of cheese, you should take a tablespoon of a fiber supplement in a full glass of water at the same time.

24

Feed Your Brain Correctly

Thanks to the pioneering work of many scientists, especially the Wurtmans, a husband-and-wife team at MIT, we now understand how our brains and our moods are affected by food. And we all know from good and bad experiences how these moods affect our lives. You have already seen how what you eat affects blood sugar and how blood sugar can affect your anxiety level. You're now ready for the graduate course in managing your mind through food.

NEUROTRANSMITTERS

Our brains, similar to every organ and tissue in our bodies, consist of cells, billions of them; in fact, there are probably more cells in the human brain than there are stars in the entire galaxy. In the brain, these cells must transmit messages from one to another that ultimately become your mood, which affects how you interact with the world. These messages go from cell to cell by what we call neurotransmitter chemicals, or simply neurotransmitters, for short. There are three neurotransmitters: dopamine, norepinephrine, and serotonin.

Dopamine and norepinephrine are the alertness chemicals. When these alertness chemicals are produced, people are more attentive, think more quickly, and, in general, are what we'd call motivated. During these periods people will often fire off ideas or commands, give a stirring speech, and take other actions, which if correctly directed can be very productive.

Serotonin is the calming chemical. Elevating serotonin acts as a brake when your thoughts are racing in all directions and you need to filter the mixed signals coming in. In short, serotonin is the opposite of the alertness chemicals; it eases the effects of stress and tension and helps you focus.

Your brain makes these neurotransmitters from two amino acids, which are the building blocks of protein. It would seem, then, that eating the correct proteins can produce the right balance of the alertness and calming chemicals.

The two amino acids are tyrosine, from which both alertness chemicals (norepinephrine and dopamine) are made, and tryptophan, from which the calming chemical (serotonin) is made.

The ancient Greeks knew that eating protein produced the alertness chemicals. Indeed, their idea that if you ate wildcat meat you'd get the prowess of the wildcat was somewhat correct. Eating protein (and a wildcat is mostly protein) yields an abundance of tyrosine, and since there is a built-in clearinghouse called the blood-brain barrier that makes it hard for tryptophan to get in, the Greek athlete

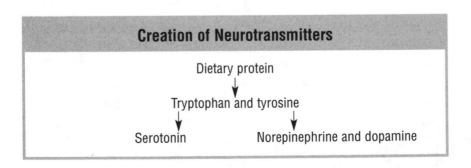

Creation of Neurotransmitters

Dietary protein

Tryptophan and tyrosine

Serotonin   Norepinephrine and dopamine

would be more alert. If he was entering a wrestling match, for example, he'd probably do better.

For tyrosine to cross the blood-brain barrier, it simply needs to be in the blood. Tyrosine, along with most other amino acids, is used readily by the brain; these amino acids readily cross the blood-brain barrier. Since there are lots of these amino acids in most protein foods, such as meat, fish, and dairy products, and even in beans and mushrooms, eating protein generally increases alertness.

Tryptophan is the least plentiful of the six essential amino acids that the brain needs. So, when protein is eaten, the amount of tryptophan that can get into the brain is limited. Suppose there are only red and black cars in the world and there are thirty black cars for every red car. Now suppose that to cross a bridge all cars must go through a series of ramps that work by alternative feed. When you look at the bridge, you'd notice that about one in thirty cars was red. In fact, if you looked for only an instant, you'd probably think there were only black cars in the whole world, and it would take awhile before you realized that some cars were colored red. That is the tryptophan problem in a nutshell. There is such an abundance of other amino acids that the small amount of tryptophan is hardly noticed. However, Mother Nature has devised a way around the tryptophan scarcity problem, which enables us to adjust our moods by eating correctly.

You've encountered the hormone insulin more than once in this book. It is responsible for the correct use of blood sugar and works by opening the door in each cell that allows in blood glucose. When insulin opens the door for glucose, it also lets in the other amino acids, except for tryptophan, which is bound to but is not a part of a special blood protein called albumin. Consequently, tryptophan doesn't tag along.

Eat a diet rich in complex carbohydrates along with appropriate protein and the blood level of tryptophan will slowly build. The other amino acids decline because they are entering all cells where they go to the manufacture of bones, muscle, skin, hair, and all the other body structures that are rich in protein. Over time, a diet that is consistently rich in complex carbohydrates will allow tryptophan to build up to a consistent level and go past the blood-brain barrier as required.

Eating for Neurotransmitter Balance

Eat protein-rich foods alone and you will notice that you are more alert and respond more quickly to mental challenges. Try eating a high-protein meal with little fat and no carbohydrates; for example, eat a chicken breast without skin, or very lean, well-trimmed beef, or a lean fish, such as flounder fillet, and no other food. See if you feel more alert and energetic in about an hour or so. Try this some evening and see if it is easier to get to sleep.

Eat carbohydrate-rich foods and you'll notice you are less stressed and anxious and more relaxed. You can focus better. In contrast to the protein meal, try a meal of only rice or pasta with tomato sauce, or beans or oatmeal. Within about an hour or so, see if you are more relaxed. Indeed, go a step further and do it in the evening and see if you fall asleep more easily.

The question becomes this: Which foods work best for you?

Table 24.1

Alertness-Promoting Protein Foods

Rating	Food Sources
Excellent	Fish, shellfish, chicken (no skin), veal, very lean beef
Very Good	Low-fat cottage cheese, skim milk, nonfat yogurt, peas and beans, lentils, tofu and other fermented soy foods
Good	Beef, lamb, pork, processed meat, hard cheese, whole milk, regular yogurt

Protein

In previous chapters you learned that fat is not good. In fact, fat will help tie up oxygen so it slows everything down; it will do the same thing here. Hence, you should always emphasize low-fat meals. Table 24.1 puts protein into three classes for the purpose of promoting alertness—excellent, very good, and good—based on carbohydrate and fat content.

Carbohydrates

Nutritionists classify carbohydrates into two groups: simple and complex. The simple carbohydrates are the processed sugars, such as table sugar, and the natural sugar, fructose, found in sweet natural foods, such as fruit. Complex carbohydrates are the starches you find in vegetables, some fruits, cereals, and grains.

The simplest way to elevate blood glucose, which in turn would elevate insulin, with tryptophan to follow, would be to eat glucose. Yuck! Not only would you not want to eat glucose, but the effect would last only a short time as your body would produce insulin in large quantities. Carbohydrate foods can be classified by their ability to produce a reasonably fast response, however, as shown in Table 24.2.

Notice there aren't any vegetables or salad ingredients listed in Table 24.2. That is because they're neutral. Their carbohydrate is delivered so slowly they don't count.

Table 24.2

Response Times for Carbohydrates

Quick Acting	Candy, cookies, pie, cake, ice cream, soft drinks, sweet syrup, preserves
Long Acting	Bread (including muffins, bagels, and so on), crackers, pasta, potatoes, rice, corn, barley, oatmeal, kasha

Eating a meal that contains both protein and carbohydrate will always power the production of the alertness chemicals. However, once your brain is producing them at its normal, optimum rate, it is not going to produce more. So, an average meal won't produce any obvious change.

In contrast, if you want to slow down and be able to focus more, a meal of pasta with tomato sauce and a side salad should be your choice.

If you want to be very alert for a morning meeting or other activity, a good meal would be a broiled flounder fillet or a piece of chicken breast. Alternatively, drink a couple glasses of skim milk or eat nonfat cottage cheese.

Test yourself. Try the obvious variations that come to mind. Eat a high-protein, low-fat breakfast with no carbohydrate foods. See how you respond. Are you more alert? Energetic? When do you run out of energy?

Eat a breakfast of oatmeal with a soy beverage and a bagel. See how you feel during the morning. Are you more relaxed? Focused? As quick to react?

Once you have determined your response level, you can start planning your meals to meet anticipated demands. In addition, if you have a late-night dinner, you might realize it is better to order pasta than steak.

Some people might read this and be tempted to run to the health food store to purchase the amino acids tyrosine and tryptophan in an attempt to bypass the food and cut to the bottom line. It won't work! Not only that, the possible side effects of taking extra amino acids, which include high blood pressure, could spell serious trouble.

THE BRAIN AND THE OMEGA-3 OILS

Any biochemical analysis of the brain proves that a brain is mostly fat. Closer analysis shows it also contains some highly specialized fats we call the omega-3 oils. In this case, "oil" is simply another word for "fat." It is important for good mental function to maintain these oils in your diet. This is not easy unless you follow some pretty important dietary guidelines that emphasize eating fish and using a sensible supplement.

Research, though far from complete, indicates that omega-3 oils are very important for brain function and vision, and their deficiency can cause mild depression and other behavioral problems. Unfortunately, it takes a long time for their levels to become sufficiently reduced for these symptoms to show up, and then they're likely to be confused with other problems. Worse, when the levels are restored, say, by diet or with supplements, it takes up to two years to build back to normal. It is just common sense to make sure you get enough from your diet, supplements, or both.

Eat cold-water fish at least three times weekly. These include salmon, freshwater trout (farm raised or caught), anchovy, mackerel, eel, herring, and tuna.

Fish oils are sold in supplement form. Some labels say EPA, or eicosapentaenoic acid. Take one or two such capsules daily.

In addition, you can take out an "insurance policy" by using a flaxseed oil supplement daily, about one teaspoon. Flaxseed oil is available in most health food stores and is also sold in capsules. A simple, reasonably inexpensive way to supplement your diet with omega-3 oils is to add a tablespoon of flaxseed oil to your high-fiber cereal daily, or to take three capsules daily.

25

Try Herbs

Our current herbal renaissance has led to serious medical scrutiny of some classic herbs, and a few of them have been proven effective. Some herbs, if used correctly, can help manage stress.

However, a misconception has emerged among herb users that must be addressed. We accept the fact that prescription and over-the-counter drugs often have unwanted side effects because they are biochemically active and alter our physiology. Herbs are no different; in fact, many of our most effective drugs—for example, aspirin—began life as herbs.

Herbs that work for a condition or symptom do so because they provide one or more physiologically active substances that relieve one or more symptoms. That means effective herbs probably have some unwanted side effects, and occasionally a person can become dependent on an herb. Dependence means that if the herb is stopped, withdrawal symptoms can appear and create a dangerous condition. Just because herbs are natural doesn't mean they can't still exert serious, unwanted side effects. Always use healthy caution.

With that in mind, the following herbs—valerian, kava-kava, and ginseng—have been proven effective, and they work to alleviate symptoms of stress.

VALERIAN

Valerian root was probably the first human tranquilizer, and its appearance in human use is lost in the fog of prehistory. As far as we know, it has been used for at least one thousand years to help people "calm down" and cope with what we modern people would call a stressful environment. As with many herbs, it can be found in copies of the *United States Pharmacopoeia* before 1940, and it first appeared around 1850.

Valerian's active and natural biochemicals work by attaching themselves to the same sites in the brain that are affected by modern medications, such as tranquilizers and mood elevators, which a doctor would prescribe for stress and anxiety. Animal research leaves little doubt that valerian is effective in helping people cope with stress and the anxiety that follows.

The dosage of herbs can be problematic because they aren't standardized as medications and vitamins are. So, the dose of valerian varies with the method of preparation. Daily use should not exceed 1.5 grams of plant material. That translates to:

- 15 to 20 drops of a 1:5 tincture in water two or three times daily;
- 1 teaspoon of root steeped ten minutes in hot water, three times daily; or
- 1 tablespoon of valerian juice three times daily.

Valerian comes with several precautions:

- Not for pregnant women.
- May cause frequent urination.
- Use caution when operating machinery.
- Never use when taking Ativan, Valium, or Xanax. Ask your pharmacist about other drugs.

KAVA-KAVA

Kava-kava is a muscle relaxant and antianxiety herb that has been clinically tested and proven effective. Kava-kava has been used for hundreds, if not thousands, of years in Polynesia. Since there is no written ancient history of this area, no one can say when its use began, but we do know kava-kava has been used as a relaxant for centuries. It is often called simply kava. Clinical studies have actually compared kava-kava to prescription antianxiety medications with reasonably equal results.

A daily dose of about 200 milligrams of kava-kava can be spread over three doses of about 65 milligrams each. The actual amount will vary according to the source, so take a 40- to 70-milligram dose three times daily and see if it helps you through a period of stress and anxiety.

Kava-kava, like most herbs, has not been tested specifically for safety in either large quantities or in normal use over long periods of time. However, its widespread employment over hundreds of years amounts to millions of human years of use with few reports of side effects. It is a physiologically active relaxant, though, and caution is appropriate when using alcohol or any psychoactive medication.

GINSENG

For millennia, ginseng has been used as a tonic to counteract stress and improve health. Since its use undoubtedly predates the first Asian medical writings, a safe bet would place ginseng as having been in active use for over twenty-five hundred years. While its actual effects are still elusive to modern medical science, its extensive use over two millennia suggests it's doing something useful.

Chinese medicine classifies ginseng as an "adaptogen." Since this doesn't comply with any standard classification in Western medicine, it's not difficult to be somewhat confused. The Chinese herbalist-physician would say that ginseng comes into its own when a person is stressed to his limits. So, its use would seem to be appropriate in our complex, competitive, and stressful society.

This indication makes sense in view of some clinical studies of ginseng and its many components. It is important to recognize, however, that ginseng provides many active compounds appropriately called genesides. Either ginseng itself or specific genesides have been shown to elicit the following physiological effects:

- Lowers blood pressure.
- Improves reaction to visual and auditory stimuli.
- Improves oxygen utilization during physical exercise.
- Reduces heart rate in physical exercise.
- Improves work output.
- Improves aerobic capacity.
- Improves mood and outlook.

The above tabulation suggests that an adaptogen is both a stimulant (improves alertness) under some conditions and a relaxant (lowers blood pressure) under other conditions. Perhaps adaptogen is an appropriate description, and over two thousand years of use is correct.

In China, Korea, and Japan, ginseng is used in tea, which characterizes its most effective use everywhere. However, in the United States, people always seek more convenient delivery and want things to work quickly. Hence, it can be found in pills, capsules, and even candies. There is absolutely no proof that these forms work or do not work, so experience must be your personal guide. When using any herb that has a history as rich as ginseng's, it is best to follow traditional use. Ginseng tea is quite pleasant and simply taking your time to drink it will have a calming effect. Take one teaspoon (1.75 grams) of dried ginseng root in a cup of boiling water twice daily. Most experts recommend drinking ginseng tea for at least three weeks; others suggest up to three months.

Ginseng is now sold in doses of from 100 milligrams to 500 milligrams as tablets, capsules, or powder. It is important to follow the directions that come with these preparations. One consistent point in the folk wisdom surrounding ginseng is that it must be used regularly for three weeks to three months to be fully effective. Therefore, it makes sense to take a smaller dose regularly than a large dose just once or twice.

Although ginseng's history indicates it is safe for most human use, it makes sense to exercise sensible caution. Common sense dictates that pregnant women should consult their doctors before using any herb or medication, even though ginseng is used by many pregnant women in Asia.

Conclusion

Stress is a double-edged sword. Without it, boredom and monotony slowly lead to mental and physical decline, but too much stress can have the same effect. Most people are challenged by pressures both at work and at home, so constant boredom isn't a widespread problem. Instead, most of us face excess mental stress, directly or indirectly leading to degenerative diseases, such as high blood pressure, heart disease, and even cancer. Like everything else, achieving the right balance is what a healthy, well-adjusted life is all about.

Setting priorities and goals in every significant part of your life is fundamental in gaining control over your environment. Prioritizing objectives provides the yardstick against which most challenges and events can be measured, allowing you to walk away from some stressors, neutralize others, and conserve your reserves for those that must be confronted head-on.

Exercise is the best and most effective way to dissipate the effects of unavoidable stress on your body. It is more than just therapeutic for a bad day; each exercise session helps your body grow stronger and more durable. The worst thing you can do is resort to stimulants, alcohol, relaxant drugs, and excessive eating to alleviate stress.

Maintaining control over stress requires that you become stronger than the stressor pulling you down. Accordingly, a healthy body is absolutely essential to maintaining your equilibrium and achieving your objectives. Sound, basic nutrition is the foundation on which all health rests; health experts don't call it preventive medicine for nothing. It only takes a little effort to eat for good health, and the dividends reaped are incalculable. Eating wisely and using sensible supplementation will help you achieve both physical and mental fitness.

Look in a mirror daily and assess what you see. Obviously, you can't pick new parents or change your genes, but you can eliminate excess flab and tone your body. Good health not only provides a longer, more fulfilling life but is vivid physical and mental proof that you can gain and maintain control of your life despite the daily stresses you face.

Index

Tables are indicated by an italicized *t*.